About the

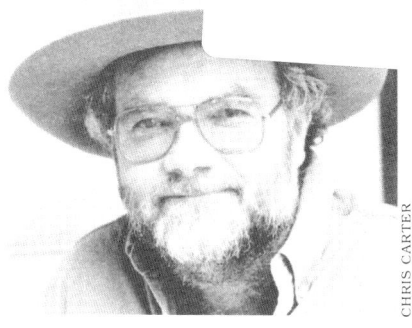

Bill 'Swampy' Marsh is an award-winning writer and performer of stories, songs and plays. He spent most of his youth in rural south-western New South Wales. Swampy was forced to give up any idea he had of a 'career' as a cricketer after a stint at agricultural college was curtailed because of illness, and so began his hobby of writing. After backpacking through three continents and working in the wine industry, his writing hobby blossomed into a career.

Swampy runs writing workshops throughout schools and communities, and is employed part-time through the Adelaide Institute of TAFE's professional writing unit. He has won and judged many nation-wide short story writing competitions, and performs his stories and songs regularly on radio, television and stage. His plays have been performed across Australia.

To discover more about Swampy's work, visit www.billswampymarsh.com

Other books by this author

Beckom Pop. 64
Old Yanconian Daze
Looking for Dad
Great Australian Flying Doctor Stories
Great Australian Shearing Stories
Great Australian Droving Stories
Great Australian Railway Stories
More Great Australian Flying Doctor Stories

Great Australian
FLYING DOCTOR STORIES

Bill 'Swampy' Marsh

ABC
Books

Published by ABC Books for the
AUSTRALIAN BROADCASTING CORPORATION
GPO Box 9994 Sydney NSW 2001

Copyright © Bill Marsh 1999, 2007

First published as Great Flying Doctor Stories *in November 1999*
Reprinted eight times
This edition first published in October 2007
Reprinted December 2007
Reprinted January 2008
Reprinted June 2008

All rights reserved. No part of this publication may be reproduced, stored in a retrieval system or transmitted in any form or by any means, electronic, mechanical, photocopying, recording or otherwise, without the prior written permission of the Australian Broadcasting Corporation.

ISBN 978 0 7333 2007 1

Cover design by Josh Durham, Design By Committee
Cover image courtesy of the Royal Flying Doctor Service
Designed and typeset in 12/15pt Granjon by Midland Typesetters, Maryborough
Printed in China by Everbest printing Co. Ltd

To Margaret and James Holdsworth,
and Jarrod Bonnici

Special thanks to

Lyn Shea for her ideas, support and enthusiasm
The Royal Flying Doctor Service and its supportive staff
Ian Doyle, Broadcaster
Angela Faraj, Public Relations, RFDS (National)
The Broken Hill Outback Residencies Program
All those who so willingly shared their stories with me.

Contents

Contributors	x
Foreword	xi
A Cordial Invitation	1
A Day at the Races	8
A Mother's Love	14
A Piece o' Piss	16
A Stitch in Time	22
A Very Merry Christmas	25
And He Survived!	27
An Egg a Day	31
And the Winner is . . .	36
And then there were Seven	39
As Full as a Boot	43
As Soft as Air	49
Born to Fly	54
Brainless	59
Break a Leg	62
Cried Duck	66
Dog's Dinner	69
Down the Pub . . . Again	73
Fingers Off	76
From Bad to Worse	81

Great Break Aye!	87
Gwen's Legacy	91
Handcuffed	93
Heaven	98
Kicking the Dust	100
Knickers	104
Love is . . .	108
Mayday! Mayday!	110
Missing	114
Mission Impossible	117
Mud Happens	120
Night Eyes	126
No Thanks!	131
Off	135
Old Bill McDougall	140
Once Bitten, Twice Shy	146
One Shot	150
Pass the Hat	153
'Payback'	158
Peak Hour Traffic	165
Pepper Steak	169
'Plonk'	174
Rabbit	178
Richmond	183
Run and Catch	188
Skills and Teamwork	190
Snakes Alive!	193
Spot on Time	197

Squeaky the Stockman	201
Stowaway	206
The Pedal Radio Man	209
The Telegram	213
The Tooth Fairy	215
There's a Hole in the . . . Drum	218
There's a Redback on the . . .	223
Touch Wood	226
Train Hit by Man	230
We Built an Airport	235
Welcome to Kiwirrkurra	239
Where's Me Hat?	242
Whistle Up	245
Willing Hands	249
You Wouldn't Read About It	253

Contributors

Great Flying Doctor Stories is based on stories told to Bill 'Swampy' Marsh by:

Joyce Anderson
Helen Austin
Bob Balmain
Joy Barton
Rosemary Chamberlain
Ben Dannecker
Maurie Denison
Ian Doyle
Jan Ende
Penny Ende
Brett Forrester
Anne Hindle
Campbell Holmes
Bob Irvine
Ray Jenner
Alf 'Bomber' Johnson
Verona Keen
Bill Legg
Geri Malone
Fred McKay
Marg McQuie
Lindsay Millar
Jack Mills
Mary Patricia Mitchell
Colin Munro
Liz Noonan-Ward
Fred Peter
Lorraine Rieck
Robert Ryan
Bruce Sanderson
Gabrielle Schaefer
Rob Seekamp
Chris Smith
Clyde Thomson
Audrey Tregoning
Penny Wilson
Maureen Woods

. . . and many others.

Foreword

Just after my last book came out I was having a cup of coffee with 'the lady down the road' (Lyn Shea). 'What're you going to write next?' she asked.

'I'm not sure,' I replied. 'Have you got any ideas?'

True to form, she had plenty, one of which was a collection of stories of the experiences people had with the Royal Flying Doctor Service.

And so began this book.

After receiving some funding from Arts SA I headed off to Broken Hill as part of a writer-in-residence program as well as to collect stories from a couple of friends of friends who worked out at the RFDS base. I was welcomed there, as I was at all the RFDS offices that I visited, with open arms and a swag of stories ready to be told.

'I'll knock this off in a couple of months,' I said.

But, friends of friends have friends of their own and before long, whenever I mentioned that I was collecting Flying Doctor stories, someone would say, 'Oh, you've got to get in contact with so-and-so. They've got a great story to tell.' So I did, and after I collected their story they, in turn, would suggest someone else who had 'an even better story to tell'.

Then amongst all this story collecting I met a bloke, Ian Doyle, who was relieving on the ABC's Sunday morning radio program, Australia All Over, and he interviewed me about the project. The response was astounding. People rang from all over Australia, wanting to tell their story; unfortunately, more than there was space in this book for. I hope that, as time goes by, I get to meet many of the people I could only get to interview by telelphone.

The stories of the contributors' experiences with the Royal Flying Doctor Service and of their triumph against the odds have been an inspiration. So sit back, relax, and allow me to introduce you to some of Australia's unsung heroes and great characters . . .

Bill 'Swampy' Marsh

A Cordial Invitation

I reckon it must have been back in about 1960 or '61, whichever year it was that copped the worst of the floods. There was this bloke, Harry, who was the Head Stockman out on Durham Downs Station. A very knowledgeable bushman he was too. Anyway, Harry and his team of stockmen had been out mustering, day in, day out, for three months straight, in woeful conditions, so when they were given a week off they decided to exercise their bushman's rite and go into Noccundra to let off a little steam in at the pub there.

'Let's get the hell out a here,' Harry called to his stockmen as they clambered up on top of the two-wheeled camp trailer, cashed up and ready to go.

Now I don't know if you've ever seen one of these camp trailers but they're massive bloody things, and they have to be. Because when you're out mustering for months on end they carry the whole kit-and-caboodle — all the food, the cooking gear, the swags, water, fuel, toolboxes, the lot. They're like a bloody huge mobile kitchen cum garage, and they've got these gigantic truck tyres on them, so huge that you'd almost have to be Sir Edmond Hillary to climb up on the tray.

To complete the picture for you, this particular camp trailer was pulled by a Deutz tractor which was driven by the camp cook, an Afghan bloke who had extremely dark skin, so dark, in fact, they reckoned that the only thing you could see of him in the dead of the night was the whites of his eyes. That's when he wasn't sleeping, of course, or praying, which was something he did quite regularly, being the extremely devout Muslim that he was. This bloke's name was Frozella, Frozella the Afghan cook.

So off this mob of stockmen went through flooded creeks, rivers and tracks and, when Frozella finally pulled into Noccundra, Harry and his workmates went straight to the pub. And that's where they spent the entire week, in the pub, except for one very important trip which Harry made. That was to the local store to buy a bottle of raspberry cordial. The reason behind that was, on their return journey they were going past an outstation on Durham Downs. And on this outstation there was a man and his wife and their three or four children and Harry had solemnly promised these youngsters that he'd bring them back a bottle of raspberry cordial, for a special treat.

As you might imagine, during that week in at the Noccundra pub, a lot of fun was had. A lot of alcohol was consumed too, which led to the usual number of stoushes. But no harm done. Anyway by the time they set off back to Durham Downs, Harry and his team were so knackered from their week's activities that not long after they'd crawled up on the camp trailer, to a man they'd fallen into a deep alcohol-induced sleep. And there, draped right up on top of the load was Harry, snug and snoring under his military overcoat, and stuffed into one of the pockets of that coat was the precious bottle of raspberry cordial.

So there they were, in the dead of the night, a few hours out from Noccundra when they hit a bump. Off came Harry. Down from a great height he fell. And when he hit the ground he was not only knocked out cold from the impact but also the bottle burst and raspberry cordial went all over him. Now, none of the stockmen realised that their boss had disappeared. Neither did Frozella. He kept on chatting away to Allah while negotiating the tractor along the muddy tracks until he reached the boundary gate.

It was while he was at the gate that Frozella did a number count and discovered that Harry had gone missing. Now the little Afghan realised that his life wouldn't be worth living if he arrived back at Durham Downs minus his boss. So with the other blokes still fast asleep, he turned the camp trailer around and drove back in search of the Head Stockman. He'd travelled about twenty miles when there, illuminated by the mud-splattered glow of the tractor lights, Frozella saw Harry laying spread-eagled on the ground, covered in red gooey stuff.

So shocked at the scene was Frozella that he sat glued to the seat of the Deutz tractor. 'Oh Allah, oh Allah,' he prayed from the safe distance, hoping for a miracle and that suddenly Harry would arise and walk. But he didn't. Harry didn't even move a muscle. This caused Frozella to conclude that Allah had instigated the accident as a punishment for all his sins. Sins that kept multiplying in Frozella's brain the longer he looked down at Harry, lying prostrate in front of the tractor.

Then the panic really set in. Without bothering to check the body, Frozella turned the camp trailer around again and raced to Kihee Station. It was there that he told the station owner's wife, Mrs O'Shea, all about his sins, and how Allah had caused Harry to fall off the camp trailer, and about how the camp trailer had run over the Head Stockman.

'Oh Missus, blood everywhere,' Frozella kept mumbling. 'Blood everywhere.'

So Mrs O'Shea contacted the Flying Doctor.

The doctor in this case was the legendary Irishman Tim O'Leary. And Tim at that particular time was attending an extremely ill patient in at Thargomindah. So when Tim got word that the Head Stockman had been run over by a camp trailer, he organised for his patient to be flown back to the Charleville Hospital so that he could go straight out to Kihee Station and see to things there. The problem being, that because of all the flooding there was a lack of suitable transport in Thargomindah.

'I'll have a go at taking yer out in me little Hillman,' the husband of the nursing sister said.

'What we need is a tractor,' suggested Tim.

'It's the best I can do,' replied the bloke.

'Okay then,' Tim said, 'we'll give it a go.'

So they jumped into the little Hillman and set off on a nightmare journey through the mud and the slush. When they weren't getting bogged, they were pushing themselves out of bogs. And whenever they came to a swollen creek they placed a tarpaulin over the radiator so that the car's engine wouldn't stall, midstream, where the chances were that they'd be washed away, never to be seen again.

Now, while the Hillman was battling its way up the track, Jack O'Shea arrived home at Kihee Station homestead and listened to Frozella's story.

'Has anyone else seen to the bloke?' Jack asked, which of course they hadn't.

So Jack spat out a few choice words then drove off in search of Harry. A couple of hours later he came across him. There Harry was, much to Jack's amazement, sitting up beside a camp fire, attempting to dry his overcoat, the one that had been soaked in raspberry cordial.

'Good God man,' Jack said, 'yer supposed to be at death's door.'

'Yer must be jokin',' Harry replied. 'There's nothin' wrong with me that a couple of Bex and a good lie down couldn't fix.'

So Jack took Harry back to Kihee and Mrs O'Shea

rang through to Nockatunga Station, where the little Hillman had just chugged up the drive.

'Look doctor,' Mrs O'Shea explained, 'Frozella's made a terrible mistake. In actual fact, the Head Stockman's got nothing more than a headache.'

After having just spent five and a half hours driving through hell and high water, in a tiny Hillman, then to be told that he'd been called out on a wild goose chase, well, it didn't go down too well with the irate Irish doctor.

'Let it be known, Mrs O'Shea,' Tim replied, 'that if ever this Frozella chap gets ill and I have to pick him up in an aeroplane, as sure as I stand here, drenched to the bone and caked in mud, I'm gonna toss him out and, what's more, from a great bloody height!'

Now news travels fast in the bush and when Frozella heard what Tim had said, he started believing that the sparing of the Head Stockman had just been a warning from Allah, and the greater punishment of being tossed out of a plane from a great height was awaiting him. Amazingly, the little Afghan didn't have a sick day for a number of years after that, not one. That was until the time he came down with pneumonia. Real crook he was. And even then he refused to see Tim O'Leary, the Flying Doctor.

'He's a gonna kill me, Missus. Allah has foretold it,' a delirious Frozella kept muttering to Mrs Corliss who was looking after him in at the Eromanga pub.

But eventually Frozella fell so ill that Mrs Corliss had to call Tim. And when he arrived in the plane, she pulled the doctor aside. 'Look, Tim,' she said, 'Frozella's locked himself in his room and refuses to let you see him.'

Now Tim had long ago forgotten the veiled threat that he'd made about tossing Frozella out of the plane from a great height. But Frozella hadn't. Not on your life. So much so that Tim had to force his way into Frozella's darkened hotel room. And when he did, the little Afghan wasn't anywhere to be seen.

Then, as Tim tells it, as he was about to leave the room he heard the faint mutter of prayers coming from under the bed. When he took a look, he saw the whites of two huge eyes, staring back at him, agape with fear.

A Day at the Races

The William Creek Races has to be the best kept secret in Australia. It's a real true-blue bush event. Seriously good fun with a dash of alcohol. What's more, it's a great fundraiser for the Royal Flying Doctor Service, held on the first weekend in April at Anna Creek Station, about eleven hours north of Adelaide.

The scene is, 'You bring your swags, we've got the nags'. That's because all the horses and camels are provided by Anna Creek Station. Along with the races it's a gymkhana affair. No bookies allowed. There's the Dick Nunn Memorial Cup, the William Creek Cup, plus all the gymkhana events — thread the needle, barrel races, and so on.

Community Service Groups, along with other volunteers, come from all over to donate their time and energy into helping put the weekend on. Ten dollars a day allows you to eat as much as you can. And when I say 'as much as you can', I mean it that way. Because if you can get it down your throat without choking, then you can eat as much as you like.

A Day at the Races

Because, I tell you what, some of that beef's bloody tough. Again, it's all donated and mainly from the next-door neighbour's property, I might add. It's cheaper that way. Why donate your own when it's just as easy to donate the bloke-next-door's? But that's the way it is out there. Things are tight. So tight, in fact, rumour has it that the only thing a local will give you is a handshake and a homing pigeon. But, mind you, they're pretty amazing when it comes to the Royal Flying Doctor Service. That's a different matter.

The big day is the Sunday. Before then, the horses and camels are put up for auction and everyone spends up big trying to buy something that might win one of the fifteen to twenty events for the day. Up for grabs are prizes and ribbons. The owners of the winning horse or camel are supposed to keep the prizes and the jockeys the ribbons but it usually happens the other way around. The jockeys in this case are mostly station people, jackaroos and jillaroos, or anyone who can sling a leg over a horse or camel.

And these young riders don't hold back. Not on your life. They go as hard as they can, so hard in fact that they sometimes get injured. So you're up there raising money for the Royal Flying Doctor Service and you have to get the Royal Flying Doctor Service to fly up to collect these people. The airstrip's graded, flares set up, kerosene tins alight, so the plane can land at night and take someone who's injured back to Port Augusta.

I remember the time in particular when one young

stockman came a real cropper. The horse shied just past the finishing post. Down come this bloke. Thump. He hit the ground like a bucket of spuds and just laid there. Motionless he was. For about five or ten minutes he didn't move a muscle and things looked real crook.

'Where's the doctor?' the cry went up.

Being a Royal Flying Doctor Service event there were plenty of doctors about but they'd all had a beer or two or three by that stage and the last thing they wanted was to face headlines reading 'Drunken Doctor Attends to Injured Rider'. So all these doctors gathered around the injured stockman. Cumulatively, well over a couple of hundred years of medical expertise was then proffered. 'Don't move him,' said one. 'Get a stretcher,' suggested someone else. 'Check his pulse,' came a voice. 'Is his windpipe clear?' another asked. 'At least get an umbrella over the bloke or he'll fry in this heat,' suggested yet another doctor. 'We'll have to get the RFDS up,' said another. 'Good idea,' half agreed. 'I don't know so much,' the other half said. 'There must be something we can do.'

It was while this verbal medical consultation was taking place that the young stockman's workmate, a big bloke he was, staggered out of the bar. 'Where's me mate Clancy?' he asked, to which someone pointed over to the gaggle of doctors standing around a prostrate figure.

So this bloke came in search of his mate. He walked over, pushed the medicos aside, took a look at his mate, and shouted 'Get off yer big fat arse, Clancy, yer nothin' but a lazy bastard.' But still Clancy didn't move. So this bloke gave him a swift boot in the bum. Thwack. In response, Clancy gave a couple of twists, woke up, got to his feet, dusted himself off, then he and his mate staggered back to the bar, arm in arm, leaving the gathering of doctors to marvel at the effectiveness of simple bush medical treatment.

Then there's the story about Phantom and his Pommie bride, Alison Tucker. How that came about was that Alison had been hitch-hiking around Australia when she ended up at the William Creek pub. Don't ask me why. It could have been fate because it was there that Phantom, the manager of Hamilton Station, caught her eye, wooed her, won her, and six months later they got married at the finish post during the William Creek Races.

A big ado that was, the full ceremony, the whole shooting match. Father Tony Redden from Coober Pedy got special permission to carry out the wedding. The William Creek Race organising committee programmed the event between the fourteenth and fifteenth race or something. Everyone was invited to attend.

Phantom called on his two best mates to be his best men, so you wouldn't reckon that there were too many secrets there. They'd all been knocking around together for years. Anyhow, when the moment arrived the three of them appeared at the top of the straight like gunslingers, dressed in black Stetsons, full black tails, waistcoats, fob watches, new RM Williams boots and cigars, the lot. It looked like something out of Gunfight at the OK Corral, especially when the wind picked up from the south-east.

As these blokes strode down the straight, everyone fell silent. You could even hear the pig sizzling away on a spit out the back. It'd been donated, a wedding gift, no doubt one of the bloke-next-door's pigs. Then as the male wedding party neared the finish post the bride and her bridesmaids arrived on the track in a Peugeot driven by the then head of the Flying Doctor Service from Port Augusta, Vin O'Brien. It was daubed with ribbons. Immaculate, it was.

Alison, who'd dressed in the William Creek pub, stepped from the Peugeot, out into the dirt, dust and flies. She looked stunning: an absolute peachy English bride, wearing a full-length wedding outfit with a parasol to boot.

Seeing as Phantom was a pretty popular bloke around the area, the ceremony had been organised to go over the loudspeaker system. So when Phantom and his mates reached the bride and bridesmaids, Father Tony stepped to the microphone and began the ceremony. Everything was going well until the Father got to the part where he read out their names . . . 'Do you Mark Spears take Alison Tucker to be your lawfully wedded wife?' he said.

At that point the service ground to a halt. There was a gasp from the outer audience. Phantom went a bright red. The bride went white with shock.

The wind dropped. The flies ceased flying. The bridesmaids turned to each other with questioning looks. The bride did the same at her bridesmaids. The bridesmaids looked questioningly at Phantom's best men. They gave a shrug. They didn't have a clue. Then everyone turned to the groom.

In his embarrassed state, Phantom leaned over to the Father. 'Excuse me, Father,' he said, 'but no one around here knows me by that name.'

'Not even the bride?' inquired Father Tony.

'Nope. Especially not the bride.'

Then Father Tony, always the professional, took up from where he left off and he said . . . 'Mark Spears, who'll be from here on known as Phantom, do you take Alison Tucker as your lawfully wedded wife?'

'Yep,' said Phantom.

'Yep, I do,' said Alison.

Then, apart from the odd smirk or two from his mates and a bit of ribbing from the outer, the remainder of the ceremony went off like a dream.

A Mother's Love

Like I said, in the days before the Royal Flying Doctor Service was set up here in Tasmania, back in about 1960, basically the only aircraft that were available for evacuations from the Bass Strait islands and other remote areas were aircraft owned by the state's two major Aero Clubs. Those clubs were the Tasmanian Aero Club, which was based at Launceston, and the Aero Club of Southern Tasmania, based at Hobart.

Now I wasn't ever a commercial pilot and I've never flown for the Flying Doctor Service, as such. I was just a private pilot who flew out of our local Launceston club back in those early days. The aircraft we were using at the time was the single-engine Auster J5 Autocar, which was a small four-seater fabric aircraft.

But the most heart-wrenching trip I ever made was after a couple of children had been severely burnt, out on one of the islands. These kids got inside a car and were playing with matches or whatever. There they were, mucking about when the vehicle exploded in flames, leaving them trapped inside. So we got the call during the night and I think it might've been Reg Munro, our Chief Flying Instructor, who flew out and brought the children back to the Launceston Hospital.

Anyway, the following day I went over to the island to pick up the children's mother. Now just before I took off I heard that one of the kids had died. The problem was that, when I picked the mother up, it was obvious that she hadn't yet been informed about the death. Remind you, I was just doing the job as a private pilot through the Aero Club so it wasn't really up to me to inform her that her son had just passed away.

But, God, I felt for that poor woman.

I reckon that there'd be nothing worse than to lose one of your own children, especially one as young at that little fellow was. So there I was flying this woman back to Launceston, knowing that her child had just died, and knowing that she hadn't yet been told about the death. And there she was sitting in the plane with me, full of a mother's concern, full of a mother's hope, full of a mother's love.

A Piece o' Piss

I wasn't working at the time so the only company I had at home, apart from the kids that is, was a little transistor radio. Now in saying that, there wasn't much to listen to around Broome in those days, other than Radio Australia. So what I used to do, was to tune into the Royal Flying Doctor Base and listen to all the telegrams, and the gossip, and in particular to the medical schedules.

The reason why I kept such a close ear out for the medical schedules was that my husband, Tony, was the Flying Doctor, and by listening in on the tranny I was able to find out when, and if, Tony was coming home. Now that might sound like a strange way of going about things but quite often he got so caught up in what he was doing that he didn't have the time to give me a ring. I mean, he might go out to a station to attend some emergency or other during the morning and end up in Perth later that night, and what's more have to stay there for a couple of days or more. You just didn't know what was going to happen. But that's how the life of a Flying Doctor was, and we adjusted to it.

A prime example was the time the RFDS pilot Jan Ende flew over from the Derby base with the Flight Sister, Ronda, to pick up Tony and go out on routine clinics around the area. They'd had a very quiet morning and Jan was flying the plane back to Broome to drop Tony off before heading back to Derby. Anyway, I was listening in on my tranny when I heard an emergency call come through. A major car accident had occurred between Fitzroy Crossing and Halls Creek.

As it turned out, what had happened was that two elderly couples were travelling in opposite directions, one coming from Darwin, the other going to Darwin. There were four or five people involved altogether. I can't remember exactly. The road wasn't in the best of conditions, which was something that I knew for a fact because Tony and I had recently travelled over that stretch and we'd smashed the cross member of our vehicle. That's how rough it was. It was dirt, of course, corrugated, with lots of potholes and bulldust.

Anyway, one of the cars had been stuck behind a road train for a fair distance. Then when they reached the only straight stretch between Fitzroy Crossing and Halls Creek the driver thought, 'Well, it's now or never.' He put his headlights on, pulled out to overtake the road train and, wham, drove straight into an oncoming car.

Of course, with so much dust about, the truck driver didn't even notice what had happened and he continued on his way. It was only when a couple of blokes from the Department of Main Roads came along that the accident was discovered. Now, luckily, there was a radio in the Main Roads vehicle and that's when the Flying Doctor Base at Derby was alerted.

So there I was, sitting in Broome listening to this drama unfolding over my trannie. I could hear the base talking. I could hear Jan and Tony in the plane. The manager from Christmas Creek Station had also arrived at the scene and I could hear him talking. They were all in contact.

It was a chilling experience, I can tell you. But the thing that I was most concerned about was just how Jan thought he was going to put the plane down on that rough and relatively short stretch of road. What's more, the plane he was flying was a Queen Air, and a Queen Air needed about 3000 feet of straight strip to land and take off.

So I was getting quite worried listening to all this drama. Terribly worried, to be honest. So much so that it eventually got the better of me, and that's when I rang Jan's wife, Penny, who was a Flight Nurse Sister back at the base, to see how she was bearing up.

'Well,' she said, as cool as a cucumber, 'there's nothing I can do about it. The best we can do is just hope.'

By that stage, some details had been radioed through about the condition of the accident victims and Jan flew the Queen Air on to Broome so that Tony could pick up whatever medical supplies he thought might be required. Meanwhile, the manager from Christmas Creek Station and the Main Roads people had blocked the ends of the straight section of road and, as vehicles were forced to stop, they got the people out to help knock down ant hills and clear the stones off the road in preparation for the plane to land.

So Tony picked up the medical supplies from Broome and they flew out to the accident scene. When they arrived Jan did a low pass-over, to check the situation out. Things didn't look good. One of the vehicles had its engine smashed back into the driver's compartment. The other wasn't much better off. What's more, the road looked a bit iffy for landing on account of both its condition and its lack of length.

Anyway, even though Jan had to negotiate some short shrubbery on his way in, he still managed to put the plane down safely. Then Tony and Ronda set to and attended the injured. And they did a wonderful job. They really did. Especially given the conditions — the heat, the dust, the flies — and taking into account that a couple of hours had passed since the accident had occurred. And under all those external pressures they didn't miss a diagnosis: fractured hips and fractured ribs, dislocations, punctured lungs, the lot. Of course, that's excluding the usual head and body injuries and so forth that go with such a horrific collision. What's more, all the accident victims survived.

But there was still one major hurdle to overcome. With so many people being injured, there was no possible way that they could fly everyone out in the

Queen Air. Now, as luck would have it, the army was conducting manoeuvres in the area and they had a Pilatus aircraft. Now the Pilatus is just a small thing so it could only evacuate two of the injured, three at a pinch. But it had one great advantage over the Queen Air in that it was a short landing/ take-off plane which made it ideal for those sorts of conditions.

By the time the Pilatus arrived, about half an hour later, Tony and Ronda had all the patients organised and ready to be flown out. Then, lo and behold, who should jump off the army plane, none other than one of Tony's old mates from his medical student days. But this was no time for grand reunions, not on your life. It was a quick handshake, a hello, then they got stuck into loading the patients into both the planes.

Now, as I said, the Pilatus was a short landing/ take-off aircraft so it got out with no problem at all. Now came the scary bit. The Queen Air had needed every inch of the road-strip to land and, with the extra weight of the patients, things looked grim. As Jan prepared for take-off he calculated that he needed to reach a speed of at least 90 knots just to get the thing off the ground.

'Here we go,' Jan said to Tony.

Then he gunned it, and they went thundering down the road. The trouble was that by the time he got to 70 knots they were rapidly running out of straight road.

'Jan,' Tony asked, 'do you reckon we'll make it?'

'A piece o' piss,' replied Jan.

But Tony reckoned that Jan wasn't looking anywhere near as confident as he sounded. He'd gone a fearful whitish-grey colour. His face had set like concrete. He was sweating profusely, and his eyes had taken on a fixed glassy stare.

'Go, you bastard, go!' Jan called, and gunned that Queen Air like it'd never been gunned before.

At 75 knots Tony knew that they were done for. At 85 knots they'd run out of road. That's when Tony ducked for cover. Then as Jan attempted to lift the plane off the ground there came the horrible crunching sound of the propellers cutting the low shrubbery to shreds.

The next Tony knew, they were in the air.

'There,' called Jan. 'I told you so. A piece o' piss.'

A Stitch in Time

We were up at Mintabie one time, Mintabie being a small opal-mining town in the far north of South Australia. Anyway, we'd just finished doing a clinic there and we were about to pile into the car to go out to the airstrip when this ute came hurtling down the road.

'Oh, my God, something terrible's happened,' I mumbled.

'Obviously some disaster or other,' replied the doctor.

Anyway, somewhere among a cloud of dust and spitting gravel the ute skidded to a halt beside us, and out from the ute jumped this bloke. He was in a blind panic, we could see that, and he starts calling, 'You've gotta help me, doc. There's been a huge fight, an' Igor's had his chest cut open. There's blood an' guts everywhere.'

'Okay,' said the doctor. 'So where's Igor?'

'I brung him along,' this bloke replied, rushing around to the back of his vehicle. 'Here he is, right here in the back o' me ute.'

So we grabbed our medical gear and shot around to where the bloke was standing and there was Igor, all sprawled out on the floor, blood everywhere, his guts hanging out, just like the bloke had said.

'Oh my God!' I gasped.

But it wasn't so much the sight of the blood and guts that made me gasp. What really did it was the mere sight of Igor himself. Because Igor turned out to be a dog. What's more, he wasn't your normal sort of average household mutt. Not on your life. Igor was absolutely huge, massive even, and without a doubt he was most surely the ugliest thing that'd ever been born into the dog kingdom.

And not only was Igor abnormally huge and abnormally ugly, he was also abnormally angry, more angry than I've ever seen a dog be angry. Even with his intestines spilling out all over the back floor of the ute, Igor still had enough anger in him to snap off your hand in one bite. No beg pardons. And that would've been no problem at all because he had teeth on him like walrus tusks which, in a subliminal flash, made me wonder just how big and angry the other dog might have been and just how ugly it might have looked, as well. That's the dog that caused so much damage to Igor, I'm talking about.

'But Igor's a dog,' I protested.

'Igor's more than a bloody dog,' the bloke replied. 'He's me bloody best mate. Got a heart o' gold, he has.'

'But we're from the Flying Doctor Service,' I said. 'We're not vets. We don't work on animals.'

'Fer Christ's sake,' spat the bloke, 'if'n yer can stitch up a bloody person, surely yer can stitch up a bloody dog.'

Now there was no way that I wanted to get within cooee of the brute, 'heart o' gold' or not. I'm not too keen on those sorts of dogs at the best of times and I made my feelings felt. But I could see that there was a flicker in the doctor's eye and I could see that he was of a different mind and, what's more, that at that very moment he was thinking along the lines of having a go at sewing Igor back together.

'Let's have a go,' he said.

There. I was right.

So, among much fear and trepidation we got the bloke to hold Igor still and I stuck a drip into him and gave him an anaesthetic. Then, when he was knocked out, away we went.

I tell you it was one of the quickest operations in the history of canine-kind. A electric sewing machine couldn't have done the job any faster. In a flash we'd stuffed Igor's stomach back up where it was supposed to go and the doctor was busy doing a frantic stitch-up job.

Then, just as the last stitch was completed and tied off, Igor started to come to. That was made obvious because he gave a guttural growl which shook the ute right down to its bald tyres.

'Let's get out of here,' I called.

So we did. We were in that car and out of there like greased lightning.

A Very Merry Christmas

One year, just before Christmas, a small bush town hospital got in contact with us. They said they had an extremely ill patient and could we fly down and transport the person back for treatment.

'It's an emergency,' they said, so we headed down there straight away.

Unfortunately, by the time we arrived, landed and drove to the hospital, the patient had died. We were about to turn around and go back out to the airport to return to base when we were confronted by some members of the hospital staff.

'Could you take the body with you, please?' they asked.

This seemed to be a strange request, and we said so. Usually, if someone dies in one of these small towns that has a hospital, and that person's going to be buried there, in the local cemetery, they go straight into the morgue awaiting the funeral.

'Is the morgue full or something?' we asked.

'Yes, in a sort of a fashion,' came their reply.

We thought this was a little odd so we asked what they meant by their morgue being full 'in a sort of a fashion'. Either it was too full to store the body or it wasn't. Fashion had nothing to do with it. And if it was full, what kind of disaster had occurred in the town? What's more, why hadn't the Royal Flying Doctor Service been notified about it?

'What's happened then?' we asked, thinking the worst. 'A plague? A bus accident, perhaps? Shootings?'

'Something like that,' they said.

'Well?' we asked.

'Well, what?' they replied.

'Well, what sort of disaster's happened that's caused the morgue to be too full to put the body in it and why haven't we been informed?'

'Look, fellers, where's your good will?' they pleaded. 'It's almost Christmas and it'd help relieve the town of a potentially disastrous situation if you just took the body back with you and we could arrange to pick it up, say, in the New Year.'

This intrigued us even more so we decided to investigate. And it was only then that the extent of the potentially disastrous situation was revealed. The staff were right. There was no possible way that the body could have fitted into the hospital morgue. Not on your life. It was chock-a-block full of the town's supply of Christmas beer.

And He Survived!

Gee, it was pretty rudimentary back in those days. Basically, the only aircraft that were available for emergency evacuations in and around Tasmania were those that were owned by the local Aero Clubs. The main one that we used at Launceston was a single-engine Auster J5 Autocar, which was a tiny four-seater, fabric aircraft. And I tell you what, things could get pretty hairy at times, especially if the evacuation was done at night.

For example, just say a call came through in the middle of the night from one of the islands out in Bass Strait. Take Flinders Island, for instance. When that happened, the Aero Club would respond and the Chief Flying Instructor, a chap called Reg Munro, would come out and hop into the little Auster. Mind you, this aeroplane had no landing lights, no navigation lights, no instrument lights, no radio. All he had for navigational aid was a magnetic compass and a torch. In actual fact, knowing Reg, he probably took two torches along, just in case the battery went flat in the first one.

So off he'd go. Now if it was a really nice, clear, moonlit night then Reg might go direct from Launceston to Flinders Island. But that would've been a very rare occurrence. More often than not it was a bit murky so he'd have to rely on getting his bearings from the various lighthouses and townships along the way.

First, he tracked down the Tamar River to the lighthouse at Low Head. Then he headed along the north-east coast over Bridport and over a few of the other small settlements along that way where he could position himself from their streetlights. From there he tracked to Swan Island which is off the north-east tip of Tasmania.

When he came across the Swan Island lighthouse Reg turned north and headed to the lighthouse on Goose Island which was just to the west of Cape Barren Island. So he tracked to that, then just kept flying north until he reached Flinders Island. By the time he got to Flinders Island, they'd have arranged some cars along the airstrip and he landed the Auster using their vehicles' headlights as a guide. Then, once he'd landed, he'd load the patient, then fly back to Launceston taking the same route.

Now the particular incident that I'd like to tell you about wasn't a night-time evacuation, thank God, but it was just one of the many that got us thinking along the lines of 'Gee, we'd better get a bit more coordinated than this.' And that's when we first went about getting the Royal Flying Doctor Service set up here in Tasmania, which was around 1960.

What happened in this case was that a call came through that a chap from Flinders Island had received serious spinal injuries after he'd been involved in either a tractor or a bulldozer accident, I'm not certain which. Now the locals knew about the Auster's limitations so they made it very clear to us that the patient was a big man. 'A very big chap, indeed,' they said. And why they made that point was because they were only too well aware of our awkward stretcher-loading technique.

Normally, what we did to get the patient into the Auster was to first strap the person tight onto the old stretcher to minimise their movement. Then we'd open the door, tip the stretcher up sideways, and sort of wriggle it inside. When that manoeuvre had been completed we'd then have to slide the stretcher forward as far as it could go until the patient's head ended up on the floor underneath the instrument panel and their feet were facing aft. That left one seat for the pilot and one seat alongside the patient, in the back of the aircraft, for an attendant.

Anyway, with this particular chap being so big, and because of the nature of his injuries, there was no way we could strap him onto the stretcher and load him through the door by tipping him sideways and wriggling him about, and so forth. That was completely out of the question.

So Reg took an engineer along with him, a chap who worked at the Aero Club at the time. Now the aircraft had a sort of turtledeck back window, if you can imagine that, where the wing is elevated and you can look straight out through the back, through the window. When they landed at Flinders Island the engineer set to and unscrewed the window, which they then removed from the aeroplane. With that done they strapped the patient onto the stretcher and eased him in through the opening and into the plane. Once the chap was settled, the engineer then screwed the window back into position. When that was completed they flew back to Launceston where they had to reverse the procedure to take the patient out.

And he survived!

An Egg a Day

Back in April 1988 I was involved in the Great Camel Race, which was a fundraising event for the Royal Flying Doctor Service. A big ado it was, too. It took two years of planning and involved almost a hundred locally bred camels and a couple of hundred people, some from all parts of the world. To take part each competitor and their support crew had to be totally self-contained food-wise, drink-wise, medical wise and otherwise, in the race on camel-back from Uluru through the desert and over to the Gold Coast. The total distance of the journey was 3329 kilometres.

There were seven of us in our team from Coonawarra in south-east South Australia, comprising the competitor and his six support crew. Originally, I went as the first-aider but before long I landed the job of truck driver as well.

Pretty organised we were too. We even took along four White Leghorn chooks — May, Colleen, Penny and Sally — who helped us out egg-wise. On our trip up to Uluru to meet with the other competitors, after we'd set up camp each night we let the chooks out to stretch their legs and have a scratch around. To start with we used to tie string onto their little ankles which, in turn, was tied to our folding chairs so that they wouldn't get away. And they were fine with that. Friendly little things, they were. They really fitted in.

Then on one particular night, I forget where we were exactly, but there was this one-eyed dog from the caravan park where we were staying. And while we were having tea we could see this dog under the truck, slinking along on his belly, eyeing the chooks off with his one eye, thinking that here was an easy feed in the offing.

'Someone's gonna have to keep a close eye on those chooks,' the cook said, half as a play on words and half seriously because, as I said, the dog only had one eye. Do you get it?

So I guess that's when it was decided that my responsibilities as first-aider and truck driver were to be expanded to include the all-important job of — Chief Chook Minder.

This added responsibility was something I didn't mind at all. As I said, the chooks were friendly little things and we'd sort of hit it off right away. What's more, as it turned out, being Chief Chook Minder fitted in well with my other jobs. See, I had a fair amount of time on my hands, because being the truck driver, what I did was to drive ahead down the track for about 10 kilometres, then wait for our competitor, Chatter Box the camel, and the remainder of the support crew to catch up.

So each time I stopped, I'd let the chooks out of their cage which was on the back of the truck and they'd wander around and have a bit of freedom, like. Still I felt sorry for the poor things, being attached to something solid, so over time I weaned them off the camp chair by tying a wee rock on the end of the string so that they couldn't run too far. Then when it looked like they were comfortable with that, I got brave and took off the rocks, which meant that they just had the strings attached to their legs. Then finally I got very brave and pissed the strings off and they were fine. They'd stick close by me, no problems at all.

As I said, I had a fair amount of time up my sleeve so, after I'd sorted out the chooks and got them settled, I'd sit back and read a book or something until everyone arrived. Then, by the time the competitor got off Chatter Box I'd have his chair ready and he'd sit down and I'd change his socks and give him something to drink. After I made sure that he was okay, he'd walk for a while because with Chatter Box being the smallest camel in the race we'd worked out that if the poor thing was to last the distance our competitor had to walk at least two-thirds of the total journey.

After everyone had left, I'd pack things up and call out, 'Hey, Penny, Colleen, May, Sally,' and the chooks would come scampering over and I'd pick them up, put them back in their cage, and off we'd go again.

They became more than animals, more than pets even. They were more like companions really because they got very attached to me, Sally in particular. At night, when we were sitting round the camp fire, if she was looking for somewhere to roost she'd perch herself on my head. That'd cause Penny, Colleen and May to get jealous and they'd come over and snuggle in beside me, a bit like the way that little children do. Thinking about it now, they kept me sane in many ways. Chooks are very faithful animals, you know, those ones especially.

Anyway, one time the chooks and I were sitting in the truck up in the channel country, about 250 kilometres out of Boulia, waiting for our rider to catch up. Boulia, if you don't know, is about 300 kilometres south of Mount Isa, on the Burke River. There I was, deeply engrossed in my book. I should've known that something was wrong because the chooks weren't keen on scratching around outside that time. Instead, they'd gone real quiet and were snuggling into me like they wanted protection. So there we were, sitting in the truck, and all of a sudden a massive drop of rain hit the windscreen.

'Wow,' I said.

I was so excited. But the chooks weren't. They started cackling and carrying on. The next thing I heard was a yell from behind the truck and when I turned around there was our rider in a real panic. He hopped off Chatter Box, ran over, and jumped into the truck with me and the chooks.

What happened next was unbelievable. I've never seen rain like it. It just poured and poured, and it continued pouring and pouring for a couple of days, non-stop, until we were stuck, true and proper. The mud was so deep that it was up to the top of the wheels of the trail bike we'd brought along with us. We couldn't go forward, couldn't go back. We were stuck, with the rain still pelting down. And believe it or not, that's the only time the chooks went off the lay. Right up until the rain came they each produced an egg a day like they knew that they had an important job to do as well.

But the rain upset them. It upset the rest of us too, mind you. I got ill. The race was called off for a while due to the conditions. Yet, true to form, after the wet, those hens took up laying again.

When we finally got to the Gold Coast there was a rumour going around that they were going to knock the chooks on the head and kill them, like. But I wasn't going to be in that, no way.

'Over my dead body,' I said.

So in the end Penny, Colleen, May and Sally were taken back to their old farm in Coonawarra where they had lots of space to scratch around in. That's where they spent their well-earned retirement, no doubt telling their chickens and their grand-chickens all about their epic journey from Uluru to the Gold Coast, and the big rain that came and caused them to stop laying. And I also hope that they mentioned me in passing too, just like I do them when I tell the story, because it's amazing just how attached you can get to chooks, those ones in particular. I still miss them. They had such loving personalities.

And the Winner is . . .

I remember back when I was working for Telecom up in the north-west of New South Wales, one time. They held this Charity Ball at a place called White Cliffs, and this ball was the culmination of some pretty vigorous fundraising activities in aid of the Royal Flying Doctor Service.

Now you know how a Charity Ball works, don't you? That's when the participants, usually young beauties, have spent a while raising money for a certain charity and they hold a ball to crown the Queen, the Queen being the person who'd raised the most money. Well, this ball was exactly like that except it was called a Golden Granny Ball. So instead of young beauties, these finalists were the more elderly, or should I say more mature, type of women. And what's more, they'd come from places like Tibooburra and Wilcannia and even maybe Cobar and Wentworth. Well, these grannies had completed their fundraising activities and arrived with their hubbies and other family members for the big Charity Ball in the White Cliffs Town Hall.

AND THE WINNER IS . . .

It was your pretty standard sort of bush show. Everyone was done up to the nines at that early stage of the night. It was a BYO affair, like. You know what that means, don't you — Bring Your Own food and grog. And I specifically mention the grog at this point because the pub hadn't set up a bar in the hall, as you might naturally assume it might. No, the publican was a lot smarter than that. His line of thinking was that when the blokes had run out of grog in the hall, they'd not only wander over to the pub to buy more supplies but they'd have a couple of swifties while they were out of sight of prying eyes — in particular, the prying eyes of their spouses. Now you can't tell me that that wasn't a stroke of economic genius, especially knowing some of those blokes, as I did.

Anyway, other than the naming of the Golden Granny there were also a number of raffles held to raise money for the Flying Doctor Service. The first prize was actually provided by the publican, and consisted of a week's free grog, food and accommodation at the White Cliffs pub. There was only one stipulation, and that was that the offer had to be taken up within the next three months, before tourist season or whatever began.

Now this was a pretty sought-after prize, especially among the blokes, if for nothing else than the free food and accommodation that you'd need after spending a day drinking the free grog. The offer of free food was viewed by most as an optional extra in this case. I don't know how many books of tickets they sold but there was a fair few because I saw them being snapped up left, right and centre.

Then just before they had the crowning of the Golden Granny they drew the big raffle. You could have heard a pin drop in that hall. I saw blokes with their fingers crossed. I saw blokes with their fingers and legs crossed. I saw blokes with their fingers, legs and everything else crossed. You'd have thought that a million dollar lottery was about to take place by the looks on some of those faces.

So the judge stepped up, dug his hand in the barrel, pulled out a ticket and said, 'And the winner is . . . blue, number twenty-six.'

And you wouldn't read about it. The bloke who'd bought the winning ticket had just been banned from the pub for six months. When this matter of technicality was drawn to the attention of the judges they got the publican over from the pub and had a confab with him. God knows why this bloke had been banned. Maybe it was for creating some drunken disturbance or other. I don't know. But for whatever reason it was, it must've been pretty bad because the publican was adamant that the offer had to be taken up within the next three months. The upshot of it all was that the winner was deemed ineligible to take up his prize and a redraw took place.

And, boy, wasn't the chap nice and dirty about it.

And Then There Were Seven

The Code One Emergency came through from Papunya, the second largest Aboriginal community in central Australia. So we hopped on the plane and flew out there. There was a doctor with us that time who'd had a lot of paediatric experience.

When we landed, the police were waiting at the airstrip. They stuck us in the back of their paddy wagon and we were rushed into the Papunya Community Clinic where we were taken in to see a sixteen-year-old girl. Two community nurses were there along with the girl's grandmother and mother. Lots of other women were gathered in and around the clinic and also a mob of kids were outside wanting to know what was happening.

The young girl was going through a difficult labour. She'd been fully dilated for a couple of hours and by the time we arrived she was getting exhausted. The contractions weren't as strong as they had been and the baby wasn't being pushed out.

It's dicey in a situation like that, going into a place

where the community nurses are familiar with everyone and are held in such high standing. You sort of get the feeling that you're imposing in some way so you don't want to tread on any toes and stuff up the delicate balance of the community's social structure. You're also careful about what you say and how you say it or else you might come across as being overly pushy which could get people's backs up.

'Oh,' I said, hinting at helpfulness, 'maybe she should go to the toilet.'

'We've tried that,' came the reply.

'Then maybe she wants to walk around,' I suggested.

'No. She's tried that too.'

We weren't getting anywhere and neither was the girl. The baby had to get out someway and, no doubt, it was getting tired as well. Then after a bit of a discussion we decided to take the girl back to Alice Springs where she could have a caesarean section.

So we got the girl up and walked her over to the clinic car, a Toyota four-wheel drive, 'troop carriers' or 'troopies' they're called. They love them out there. They're ideal vehicles because there's so much room in them. You can easily fit a stretcher in the back if necessary. But in this case the girl got in the front along with the grandmother who was coming back with us, to keep her company. We hopped in the back and then we were returned to the airstrip. Then just as the young girl was being helped up the stairs into the plane I said to the doctor, 'Oh, I'll get the obstetric kit out just in case.'

There were two pilots in the plane that day, our

senior Royal Flying Doctor Service pilot and one who was on a Mission Aviator's Scholarship. They're a separate group of pilots who work for the Mission Aviation Fellowship and they do a lot of community runs in the mail plane, picking things up and dropping things off to the remote communities. The MAF were getting a new aircraft, one of the Pilatus planes, so their pilot had come along as part of his training.

Anyway, because of all the control and instrument checks and so forth, it takes about five or ten minutes for the plane to get ready for take-off. And during that time one of the jobs that the pilot has to do is to call flight control and notify them of the POB which registers the number of people who are on board the aircraft. While the pilot was doing all that the girl had four or five contractions and it became pretty obvious that she was going to have the baby much sooner rather than later.

After we'd taken off, the girl had a couple more strong contractions. We were up about 15 000 feet at that stage. I remember that the grandmother was in one seat, the doctor was in a seat, there was a crib on the back stretcher, the girl was on the other stretcher, and I was in another seat with the headphones on.

'Oh,' I said to the pilot, 'I think we're going to have a baby so I'll take the headset off for a while.'

Then just as I did, the girl gave a much stronger push so I thought that I'd better have a look; which I did and I could see about a 20 cent size of the baby's head being pushed up.

'We might move grandmother to the front seat so we have more room,' I said, thinking that by five pushes this baby would be out.

Then the doctor said, 'If you deliver the baby, I'll look after it.' Like I said, she'd had a lot of paediatric experience.

'Okay,' I replied.

So I got grandma out of the way pretty quick smart and grabbed the obstetrics gear and got the clamps and the oxygen ready. And then the baby was born. I delivered the baby. A little baby girl. It was amazing. And after I rugged up this beautiful little baby girl, I put the headset back on.

'We've just had an addition,' I announced to the pilot. 'You'll have to amend the POB.'

'Wow,' he said, 'I've been with the RFDS for seven years now and this is the first time I've ever had to amend the POB.'

Then he notified flight control. 'Flight control. Amended POB. We now have seven POB.'

Even the air traffic controller, a normally dry, quiet and emotionless voice over the airways, as they all seem to be, well, he came back on and he was also really excited. 'Yeah,' he said. 'Congratulations.'

So the baby was born and everything was fine. There was hardly any mess at all. But it was such a thrill to do it and what's more to be able to say that 'we'd done it in midair'. It was just amazing. There we were, up at 15 000 feet. We were all so excited, the young girl, the doctor, me, the two pilots and, of course, grandma. Grandma was over the moon.

As Full as a Boot

No doubt you've heard of the term 'as full as a boot'. Well, here's a story that'll take some beating. It's about a Padre who went one better.

It happened back in the Christmas of 1937 when, after a stint of work on a station up in the middle of Cape York, a stockman, a real gentlemanly cove he was, came down to Normanton to celebrate. Now this type of celebration was, and still is, a bush ritual. After a group of stockmen have been out living and working in cattle camps for months on end, as soon as the mustering season is over they take a break and head straight for civilisation, and in particular to the nearest watering hole, there to celebrate.

Anyway, along with his mates, this chap arrived at the National Hotel in Normanton determined to enjoy himself. And as occasionally happens in these situations, he got a bit carried away. Well, more than just a bit, really. He overcelebrated to such an extent that when he decided to go to bed, he encountered great difficulty in climbing the two flights of stairs leading to his second storey-room. But patience is a virtue and he awkwardly edged his way upwards, step by precarious step, much to the admiration and encouragement of his mates.

Given the condition this fellow was in, he did a sterling job. That is until he was about to take the final step in that almost 'Hillarian' climb to the summit. As he turned to wave to the cheering crowd below, a minor mishap of judgment occurred and, lo and behold, back down the stairs he came, 'Thump . . . Thump . . . Thump', until he reached the bottom and there he stayed, unconscious and injured.

After the unfortunate accident, the publican got in touch with the Australian Inland Mission at Cloncurry — the AIM being the organisation that pioneered the Royal Flying Doctor Service — saying that the chap was in real trouble at the foot of the stairs.

'Looks like the poor bloke's injured his noggin and broke his shoulder bone,' the publican explained.

Now this was the first real 'Flying Doctor' trip that the particular Padre in question had gone out on. Normally he was a Patrol Parson with the Presbyterian Church who, in turn, ran the Australian Inland Mission. And it was his job to cover the area from Birdsville to Normanton and beyond by road, that's if you could describe some of the bush tracks that he travelled over as being roads. In actual fact, he virtually lived in his truck, covering hundreds of miles each year, christening bush children, installing pedal wireless sets, and so forth. John Flynn used to travel with him quite a bit.

Anyway, as this clergyman prepared to get on the plane, the doctor picked up on his apprehension.

'Padre,' the doctor said, 'don't worry. This is just a plain evacuation. We'll go out there, collect this fellow, and bring him straight back to Cloncurry. All will be hunky-dory.'

With those words of assurance, they clambered into the small Fox Moth 83 Ambulance aeroplane. After turning the propeller, the pilot jumped into the outside cockpit and prepared for take-off.

Now the Fox Moth 83 was by no means an aeroplane designed for passenger comfort. It only had enough room for two seats, a stretcher and the doctor. What's more, it was held together with little more than wood, cloth, string and wire. So they set off at top speed, which was about 80 miles an hour, in the old money; about a four-hour trip it was.

When they arrived in Normanton they headed straight for the National Hotel, fully expecting to find this chap still laying at the bottom of the stairs. But nothing was going to get in the way of this stockman's big occasion. This was his big night. It was his ritual and nothing was going to curtail his celebrations, not even head injuries, nor concussion, nor shoulder injuries. Nothing! Somehow he'd gained his second wind and had managed to find his way back to the bar.

Now this chap proved to be a big man of around 15 stone, if not more. Quite a 'bush gentleman' he was, in his own sort of way, and one who could tell cattle-camp yarns by the dozen, which he seemed more intent on doing at the time than returning to Cloncurry to get his injuries seen to. But in the end four mates got him into a truck and they drove him out to the airstrip.

But getting this chap out there was only part of the fun. Like I said, he was a solid lump of a man and it took some wangling to get him into the Fox Moth and fixed up in one of the seats in the cabin. When that was done, the doctor clambered in, followed by the clergyman who sat beside the stockman. The pilot spun the propeller, the plane sparked into action, then he jumped into the outside cockpit and they prepared for take-off.

'Just keep an eye on the patient, Padre,' the doctor said, and they took off, heading back to Cloncurry.

As I said, it was a good four-hour trip, longer when there's an extra 15 stone on board. There they were, halfway to Cloncurry, and they were flying over Donor's Hill when the big stockman made it known that he'd received the urgent call of nature. His exact words won't be quoted. All I'll say is that the stockman used his own particular style of vernacular to get his point across in a crystal clear manner. The rest is up to your own imagination.

Naturally, the Fox Moth 83 didn't have the facilities to cater for such an exotic exercise. But that wasn't going to inhibit the stockman. As enterprising as he was, he took off one of his riding boots. Out it come, and he proceeded to fill the boot. Then after the stockman had filled the boot, he stood it up on the floor next to the

Padre. Now if that didn't give our good clergyman a shock, worse was to follow. The stockman then removed the other boot, the left one it might have been, and proceeded to fill that one up as well, or nearly up.

'Ah, there, that's better,' he sighed and calmly stood it up beside the other one, right next to the Padre's seat.

So there was the Padre, watching these two boots jiggle precariously about on the floor of the vibrating aeroplane when the voice of the pilot crackled through the speaking tube from the outside cockpit. 'Hold on tight, fellows,' he said, 'we're going to strike some rough turbulence over these Cloncurry hills.'

That really threw the Padre into panic. He took a look at the stockman. Then he took a look at the jiggling boots. Then he took a second look at the stockman. But the stockman didn't seem too perturbed about the matter so the clergyman was forced to take things into his own hands, so to speak, and as they flew through the turbulence over the Cloncurry hills, he steadied both boots to keep them from spilling all over the place.

They finally landed in Cloncurry where the ambulance was waiting. As soon as they came to a stop, four husky men helped lift the bulky, injured patient out of the plane and into the ambulance.

'See you later, Padre,' the doctor said as he jumped in the back of the ambulance, and off they dashed to the hospital, leaving the Padre behind.

So there he was, this Padre, standing out on the airstrip, wondering how he was going to get home when it suddenly dawned upon him that he was still hanging onto these two filled stockman's boots.

He must have looked a rare sight because the pilot appeared not long after, and didn't he have a chuckle. 'Well,' he laughed, 'I've heard of the saying "as full as a boot" — but, Padre, I reckon you might have gone one better there!'

As Soft as Air

It was just one of those nights that you really didn't need to go out flying in, especially if you were a pilot like I was. The weather was bloody abominable. It was the middle of the wet season. Thunder-storms were everywhere.

But around nine o'clock there was a call from Balgo Hills Mission, which is out across the desert, halfway between Alice Springs and Derby. Believe it or not, a chap by the name of Father Hevern ran the mission, a terrific guy he was. Anyway, they had a patient who was deteriorating rapidly.

So the doctor called me. 'Look,' he said, 'will you go?'

'Yes,' I said. 'Of course I will.'

And so I set off with the doctor and a nursing sister. Like I said, the night was exactly as predicted. The weather was foul; thunderstorms were everywhere.

It might sound a bit rudimentary but, although radar was available at that time, we were nowhere near getting it in the Queen Air that I was piloting. So

I adopted my usual technique of flying under those types of conditions and I navigated by the intensity of the lightning. That meant getting my belly down in the weeds, as the flying term goes, down to about 3000 feet, under the base of the cumulonimbus which were around 5000 to 6000 thousand feet. Then I'd wait for a bolt of lightning. That wouldn't take long.

When the lightning struck, it'd burn a photo imprint or impression on the back of my retina which gave me a bloody good idea of what was up ahead. So I just took the line from the lightning and flew in that direction until I hit another lightning strike, then on to another, and another, and so forth, and I kept on steering around the columns of rain where the most severe turbulence was.

As I said, it's called navigating by the intensity of the lightning, and it works. Mind you, we took a bit of a bloody hammering at times but it was the safest way to go.

On this particular night we wound our way through the thunder-storms, the down drafts and severe turbulence for nearly two hours. It was a pretty horrendous ride for everyone concerned. Not even the doctor or the nurse had much to say to me. Either they were too scared, or they were sick, or they just figured out that I had a few other things on my mind, which of course I did.

See, other than negotiating the foul weather there was also another problem I had to be wary of out in that area. It's what's called 'jump-up' country, a flat mesa-type landscape where high steep-sided rock plateaus just jump up in front of you. Balgo Hills Mission is a typical example. Balgo sits on top of a rocky plateau. It's quite impressive really. The only thing is that if you undershoot you'll fly straight into the side of a cliff.

So I got close to Balgo. But I still couldn't see it. They'd radioed and said they'd have the basketball court lights on but I couldn't even find them. Then as luck would have it, when I flew over where I thought the place should've been, I caught a glimpse of the mission down through some broken cloud. So I did a circuit, came back round, and lined myself up on final approach.

Now, on final approach, a pilot's technique is to look at the end of the runway and if the lights are getting further apart it means that you're getting too high and if they start to join together then you're obviously getting too low. And it was pretty important that I got the approach right this night because, as I said, if I didn't I could well fly smack-bang into a cliff face.

I set myself up on final approach all right. There was some pretty severe turbulence. The windscreen wipers were belting away, and I was sitting there glued to the lights along the runway. Then as I prepared to land I noticed that the runway appeared to be getting shorter, and I'm thinking, 'What am I seeing here?'

So I tried to analyse what my brain was telling me and, while that was going on, the runway's getting progressively shorter and shorter and more and more lights are disappearing up ahead of me. Suddenly, only about half of the lights were visible. Then less than half.

'To hell with this,' I thought. 'I've come this far, I've got to land.'

So I thumped the aeroplane across the threshold, banged it on the runway and as I did, the remaining runway lights completely disappeared. I couldn't see a thing. Not a thing.

Then it struck me. What was happening was that a thunderstorm was sweeping in and a torrential wall of water was working its way down the runway. By the time we were rolling to a stop, the runway lights on either side of the wings had vanished. You couldn't see them. That's how heavy this sheet of rain was. You couldn't have heard yourself scream inside the aeroplane from the intensity of the rain.

So we just sat there in the middle of the airstrip waiting for a slight break in the downpour and I called the doctor up and I put it to him. 'In view of the intense nature of this trip,' I shouted, 'if there'll be no dramatic improvement by transporting the patient back to Derby tonight, we should look very closely at overnighting here in Balgo and seeing how the weather is tomorrow morning.'

Well, that was duly noted. Then when there came a bit of a break in the rain, I managed to turn the aeroplane around and taxi back to the holding area where the doctor and the nurse disembarked and were rushed off to attend to the patient. After they'd gone, I did the things that I had to do then waited until someone came back and transported me into the mission.

So there I was, as it happened, in a little room at Balgo Hills Mission. The very same establishment that was run by Father Hevern. I suppose, in retrospect, it must've been a small dining room or something. I was totally by myself. By this time, it was around eleven o'clock at night. And I was sitting there reflecting about how narrow the margins of error got on the way out, and contemplating the horrors of a return flight to Derby that very same night, when I received this premonition — a spiritual experience, you could even describe it as.

A nun quietly opened the door behind me. As soft as air, she walked around and looked straight into my eyes. Then, without saying a word, she placed a bottle of Queen Ann whisky and one glass in front of me, walked out and closed the door behind her.

Born to Fly

Jim, the base director from Derby, phoned one night and said, 'Listen, Jan, we've got a bad one up at Kalumburu Aboriginal Mission.'

'What's up?' I asked.

'A guy's been run through by a bull's horn and pinned against a fence post.'

'Oh, gee, Jim,' I replied. 'Penny and I have got to go to Kalumburu at six tomorrow morning to do a clinic. Can't the patient wait?'

'No,' he said. 'The patient's dying.'

'Okay,' I said. 'We're on the way.'

Mind you, as well as being the Royal Flying Doctor Service's Flight Nurse, I was also married to Jan and six months pregnant with Dan at the time. Anyway, we rushed out to the airport and jumped into the Beechcraft Queen Air. By that time it was about nine at night.

The weather itself wasn't bad, but it was the middle of the dry season. That's when all the burning off takes place and, to make matters worse, the prevailing easterlies had brought in a mass of smoke and dust across the Northern Territory. So once I was at cruise level, I could hardly see the ground. Still, it was something that I knew I'd encounter. I'd actually mentioned it to Jim during the call — the possible complete lack of horizontal visibility due to the low-lying smoke, especially when I came in to land.

'Don't worry about that,' Jim had said. 'I'll get them to turn on the lights of the basketball court.'

As you might imagine, with the whole of the outback being dotted by fires, the lights of one basketball court weren't going to make a scrap of difference. What's more, it's bloody uncanny the way those fires seem to run in lines just like streets lights do. You'd swear black and blue that there was a town or a settlement down below. So all I really had to rely on was my previous flying experience throughout the area.

I hadn't mentioned my concerns to Jim, though. 'Thanks, Jim,' was all I'd said at the time because my mind was already mulling over another problem that I was afraid we'd run into. And I'd been right. Not long after we took off, we lost HF radio contact because the Asian radio stations were jamming the airways. They'd blown us right out of the air. For all intents and purposes we'd disappeared off the edge of the planet. No base. No bugger-all.

Still, I kept on track and heading until we eventually found Kalumburu. Now most people who fly in there will tell you that Kalumburu's a pretty risky place to negotiate because it's shaped like a dish surrounded by hills. At night some of the pilots get quite edgy about it. So we flew over the top and I caught a sighting of the mission down through the smoke. But, because of the prevailing conditions, there was no bloody way in the world that the horizontal visibility was going to permit us to see it at a low-landing level. It was like an extremely thick fog down there.

But, as luck would have it, there was some moon this night so I went back, right up over the Bonaparte Gulf and let down over the water, down to about 500 feet. Then I followed the moon path up a creek that led to the threshold of the runway. Right opposite the threshold of the runway I knew there was a bend in the creek. So I flew up there with the moon behind me, turned left at the bend and figured that the runway was dead ahead.

While Jan was doing that I'm sitting there knowing what's ahead. And I know that at the other end of the airstrip there's a great big mountain, a massive pointed lump of rock. As I said, I'm about six months pregnant at this time and I've got my hands tucked underneath my safety belt so that I can't touch anything because I'm getting particularly anxious and I'm starting to climb backwards up the seat. I don't know if you've ever climbed backwards like that, but it's quite unnerving because what you're trying to do, in effect, is to remove yourself as far as possible from the point of contact.

Throughout all this, Jan's still driving on with his eyes glued into the white smoke-filled air. He's nice and cool and collected. He's a particularly calm sort of pilot, just a natural. And I'm saying to him, 'Put the lights on, Jan. Put the lights on. I want to be able to see what's going on up ahead.' This is through the thick smoke, like. So Jan finally said, 'Oh, all right.' And he put the lights on and it's like a total nothing, nothing but a blanket of thick white. You can't see a bloody thing. At this point I'm terrified.

'All right,' I shouted. 'Turn the bloody lights off.'

So I did. I turned the lights off. By this time I reckon that I'm lined up for the runway. I just had to be because I got the turn of the creek right. The gear's down by this stage, half flap out. I still couldn't see a bloody thing. A total white-out, like Penny said. So I just keep flying the heading. 'Fly it. Fly it,' I'm saying to myself.

Then, like a flash, right before my very eyes, the first of the runway lights come into sight. Bang, the wheels hit the ground, just like that. We'd landed. We were down. We were on the runway.

So we picked up this wretched guy, the one who'd been run through by the bull's horn.

And he wasn't too bloody happy either, I can tell you. So we loaded him on board. By this stage, just about every bloody air radio station in the country is calling for us. 'Foxtrot. Delta Victor. Foxtrot. Delta Victor. Do you read me?'

It's now two hours out and nobody's heard 'boo' from us and they can't contact Kalumburu Mission anyway because the radio is out and there were no telephones in those days.

When we took off again I climbed out of Kalumburu and took the Queen Air to the highest bloody altitude it could get to, in an attempt to clear up the airways and get some range into the signal. I even tried to raise somebody on the higher VHF frequency instead of the more usual HF. There I was, calling, calling and calling, and still no bastard wanted to know me.

While Jan's doing all that, he's having some oxygen so that he can keep flying without too many problems and I'm giving the patient oxygen to keep him going. Then I'm giving me and the baby-to-be some oxygen.

Jan eventually got us out of there and back home where we delivered the patient safely. But even now Jan and I reckon that it was because of the excitement and the rush of adrenaline going through my body on that particular night, it's why our son, Dan, was born wanting to fly; which was something that he went on to do. He became a pilot, just like Jan. What's more, he still flies, right up to this very day.

Brainless

You meet some drongos in this game. You really do. Just take the fellow who wanted to go from Adelaide to Cairns. He glanced at the map. 'Ah yes,' he said, 'the shortest way is straight up the Birdsville track.'

So he set out in the middle of summer in his four-cylinder rust-bucket. He had no spare petrol. No spare water. One baldy spare tyre. No supplies. Nothing. Anyway, he got up towards the north of South Australia and the car broke down.

'Bugger,' he said, and sat there wondering what to do.

Then somewhere he remembered hearing that if you break down in the outback, rule number one is to wait with your car. So he waited . . . for the first day, the second day, the third day. By this stage he was getting a bit thirsty. And during the intercourse of these thirsty feelings he looked out over the flat shimmering landscape, and the deeper he looked into the shimmering the more it looked like there was a lake out there, away in the distance.

'There's a stroke of good luck,' he said, and hopped out of his car and set off, walking towards the lake.

The strange thing was, though, the further he walked towards the lake, the further the lake moved away from him. So at the end of the fourth day he concluded that the lake must have been one of those optical illusion things, and he decided that he'd better go back to his car.

He was surely blessed because it was a miracle that he found his vehicle. Still and all, by that stage he was absolutely perishing. It then struck him that the only water he was likely to find in a place like this was the stuff in the radiator. So he tapped the radiator. Now the radiator had anti-freeze in it, and what he didn't know was that anti-freeze contains ethylene glycol. And one of the side effects of drinking ethylene glycol is that it could well cause brain damage.

Anyway, not too much later a car came along and took him into Birdsville where he went straight to the pub and commenced oral rehydration. At that stage the Flying Doctor Service was called and we flew out to Birdsville where we gave him some intravenous rehydration. To give you some idea as to how severely dehydrated this fellow was, he was given three litres of fluid intravenously to get just one millilitre of urine out of him.

Later on, in Charleville Hospital, when he asked if there were any side effects caused by drinking radiator water, I explained that unfortunately the radiator had anti-freeze in it and that anti-freeze contains ethylene glycol.

'And what's the problem with that?' he asked.

'The main side effect,' I said, 'is that it could well damage the brain.'

'Gawd,' he said, with a worried look, 'what do yer reckon the chances of me getting brain damage might be?'

I must say that it was a struggle to keep a straight face. I mean, you'd have to be brainless in the first place to attempt to drive across one of the most unforgiving parts of Australia, in the middle of summer, in a vehicle that wasn't in any fit condition to do so, without spare petrol, water or food.

So I said to the chap, 'It's my opinion,' I said, 'that in your particular case, there'd be Buckley's chance of brain damage occurring.'

'Who the hell's Buckley?' he replied.

Break a Leg

Now I might get these couple of blokes into strife here if I mention their real names, so let's call the pilot 'Jack' and the doctor 'Don'. Anyway, the pilot who's Jack in this story was the same bloke who taught me to fly. There's a hint. And the doctor is also well known, especially around these parts. There's another hint. But I'd better not mention their true names, like I said, just in case.

One night Don got an urgent call to go out to a seismic camp where a chap had reportedly been bitten by a snake. These seismic people were doing the survey work in preparation for oil rigs to move in. There were about thirty or so men in this particular camp.

Jack was a spot-on navigator, one of the best I've ever seen. So he stoked up the Navaho and they flew to Quilpy. That way may sound like the long way of going about it, but it's a far surer way of finding someone out in the never-never than to fly to a known point then bear another heading. It shortens the distance and lessens the error.

So out they flew in the dead of night to find this camp, and when they came across it these seismic blokes were as disorganised as buggery. They were still running around trying to light up the bloody airstrip. So Jack circled the Navaho around for a while until he could get a good sighting of the runway. Then, low and behold, just as they were about to touch down one of the idiots aimed a spotlight fair in Jack's eyes, blinding him.

'The plane musta landed itself,' Jack has since told me.

Anyway, they landed safely, and when they taxied back to these seismic blokes they discovered that the whole mob of them were as drunk as skunks.

'Which one of youse is the one that's been bitten by the snake?' Don asked.

I don't know if these blokes were just playing funny-buggers or not but they were so under the weather that they reckoned they'd forgotten which one of them had been bitten. Now this sort of antic didn't go down too well with either Jack or Don, no way, not even when these idiots grabbed a chap and stripped him off and started looking for a snake bite.

'Listen,' said Don, 'if you buggers aren't sick in the head now you certainly will be tomorrow.'

And, boy, didn't he gave them a fair sort of rev. He

told them that while he was out here buggerising around there could be an horrific accident somewhere else, a life and death situation, where he was badly needed. And this is what I impress upon people, station people as well. Don't go calling the Flying Doctor out for a sore toe or a bloody broken thumb or something like that, especially if you can get the patient out in a light aircraft or motor car yourself. The Flying Doctor Service is there for emergency life-threatening complaints. They're not a bloody flying hospital factory. So, anyway, as you might imagine, both Jack and Don were pretty riled up about this pack of idiots.

Well, Jack was telling me that when he taxied down the other end of the strip to take off, he saw red. So when he turned around, he opened both taps up on the Navaho. And as she gathered speed, there were all these blokes still drinking and skylarking about on the airstrip, right in the middle of his take-off path.

'Bugger it,' he said to Don. 'I'll teach these blokes a lesson.'

So he lined them up with the plane and aimed the headlights straight at them. Blinded them just like they'd done to him. They couldn't see a damn thing. All they could hear was the drone of the Navaho bearing down upon them at a great rate of knots.

Jack reckons that he's never seen the like of it. There was this mob of drunken seismic blokes, all pushing each other out of the way, hitting the deck, tripping over themselves and diving for cover, left, right and centre, screaming and yelling.

Then as the Navaho roared over the top of them Don yelled out, 'Break a leg, you bastards, break a leg.'

Then they flew off into the night.

Cried Duck

I'm not sure if you should publish this but, just in case you do, I'll change the people's names in an attempt to protect the guilty.

My pilot, Joe, and I used to fly around the outback for the Royal Flying Doctor Service in a Dragon DH 84 plane. There wasn't much to the old Dragons really, seeing that they were made out of little more than wood, rag and string. Still, being built that light gave them one great advantage — and this did happen occasionally. If ever you needed to come in for a crash landing, you could put the plane down between a couple of trees that were close together. Now that'd wipe the wings off but, more importantly, you'd come to a fairly soft and safe halt.

But perhaps something of a more realistic concern was that, if you blew an exhaust gasket in one of the engines, the chances were that it'd catch fire. See, the Dragon had two engines, each with its own separate fuel tank. So if you blew a gasket in one of them, to save going up in flames, what you had to do was to throttle the offending engine right back which, in turn, caused you to lose ground speed. Mind you, it also put a big strain on the working engine and used up a lot of fuel in its tank as well.

Anyway, whenever Joe and I flew across the bottom of the Simpson Desert, we'd track along the Cooper Creek. The reason for that being, given the right season and with enough water about, more often than not there'd be large numbers of ducks along the creek. So Joe and I would keep an eager eye out and wherever we saw a promising place I'd call up Ted, the radio operator, back at the base.

'Look, Ted,' I'd say, 'I think we've blown an exhaust gasket in the starboard engine and we'll have to put down and take a look at it.'

'Okay,' Ted'd say. 'Please give your location just in case you need us to send someone out to get you.'

Which I'd do. Joe would land on a suitable clay pan. Then we'd take a quick look at the exhaust gasket, find that there was nothing wrong, radio Ted back and tell him that we're okay and we'll only be delayed for a while, then go and shoot some ducks for dinner.

Anyway, this particular day we were heading across the Simpson Desert at about 5000 feet. That's about as high as you could get a Dragon to fly in hot weather, and we had a forequarter of beef on board which we'd picked up along the way, legally mind you. And, lo and behold, we blew an exhaust gasket, in real life.

So Joe throttled the engine back and sagged the Dragon down to about 500 feet. Then to lighten the load we chucked the bloody forequarter of beef out and hung the plane in at between 400 and 500 hundred feet.

'Things don't look too good,' Joe said.

'Okay,' I said. So I called up the base on the radio. 'Ted, we're in a lot of strife out here,' I said. 'We've blown an exhaust gasket and we might have to put down.'

'What did you say?' he asked.

I said, 'We've blown an exhaust gasket and we might have to put down.'

'Oh right-o,' he replied, all excited, 'so it's duck for dinner again, is it?'

Then he went off the air.

Dog's Dinner

A few years ago there was this fellow out on a station who'd somehow got his hand caught in a piece of machinery and had lopped off one of his fingers. Amputated it, like.

So we got the call from this fellow; pretty laid back about the accident he was. Like most bushies, real laid back. 'Just lost me finger, doc,' he said. 'What do yer reckon I should do about it?'

'Look,' said the doctor, 'just put a bandage around the stump to stop the bleeding. When that's done get your finger, the missing one, wrap it in a tea towel which is packed with ice and we'll see if we can attach it when we get out there.'

'Ah, doc,' replied the fellow, 'me finger's pretty well, yer know, stuffed as far as I can see. It don't look too good at all.'

'Yeah, that may well be the case,' said the doctor. 'But, still and all, grab the finger, put it in a tea towel packed with ice and when we get out there we'll have a good look at it. Right?'

When we landed at the station where the fellow lived, way out it was, he sauntered over to the plane. One hand was bandaged up around the stump and he's got a tea towel in his other hand. Both the bandage and the tea towel were soaked through with blood. A real mess, it was.

So we got out of the plane. 'G'day,' we said. 'How yer doing?'

And he said, 'Oh, not real flash.'

Then we asked if we could have a look in the tea towel, just to see how bad the severed finger was.

'Okay,' he said.

As I said, this fellow had one hand covered in bandage and he was carrying the tea towel containing the severed finger in the other hand, making things a little awkward for him. Most of the ice had melted, which made it even worse. So when he went to pass over the bloodied tea towel it slipped out of his hand. Before we could catch it . . . 'plop', it came to land on the dusty ground.

Now, that wasn't too bad. But with it being a station there were stacks of working dogs around the place. And all these dogs were kelpie-blue heeler crosses and they all looked the same and they all hung around in packs of about ten or twelve, gathered around the place.

What you've got to realise at this point is that on these stations they keep their working dogs fairly lean. They don't like to overfeed them. That way they've got more stamina when it comes to mustering the sheep or cattle. Now these dogs can smell a free feed from about a kilometre away, and there was a pack of these kelpie-blue heeler crosses hanging around nearby.

Anyway, just as we were about to lean over and pick up the bloodied tea towel containing the mangled finger, one of the dogs shot out from the pack and started ripping into it, tearing it to shreds. We attempted to take the tea towel from the dog but, in a frenzy of hunger, it let us know in no uncertain terms that there was no way it was going to give it up. It was in no mood to have a free feed taken away from it.

In a flash the dog had munched the tea towel to shreds, then it scampered back into the safety of the pack. So we searched for the severed finger among the shredded tea towel but couldn't find it, which left us to assume that the dog had swallowed it. The problem was, with a pack of ten or twelve of these dogs looking exactly the same, we had no hope of working out which one had just eaten this poor guy's finger. Neither did he. He took a look at the tea towel strewn across the ground, then a look at the pack of dogs.

'Beats me which one it was,' he said with a shrug of his shoulders.

'What can we do now?' we were thinking. 'Don't panic. Okay, we can knock these dogs out, open them up one by one. Then, when we find the finger, we can assess the situation and take it from there.'

But the fellow must have read our minds. He gave the remnants of the tea towel a bit of a kick with his riding boot and said, 'Ah, fellers, take me word fer it.

The finger was pretty much stuffed anyways. What's more, there's no bloody way yer gonna cut open any of my dogs just to look fer me missing finger. I got nine of the buggers left, anyways.'

Down the Pub . . . Again

Mate, my story concerns my sister and my brother-in-law. They've since been divorced, but when all this went down they weren't getting along real well. What's more, my brother-in-law was spending a hell of a lot of time in the various pubs around the place. He had a forestry business, a forestry business where he was a logger. But at this particular time the weather had been too rough for logging out in the forest so he'd taken his team into Cairns, where they were working in a shed.

Then one day around lunchtime my brother-in-law decided to go off, up into the forest, and check out the site where they'd been logging, just to get some idea of how long it'd be before they could get back out there, like. Now the particular camp he wanted to visit was about 140 miles north of Cairns, out on the Cooktown road, way back in the forest.

Anyway, as was normal with my brother-in-law, he jumped into his vehicle and off he went without telling anyone. And when he got up there, down came the rain like you wouldn't believe and a flash flood locked him in.

'Bugger,' he said, 'I'll be stuck up here for days now.'

Then he started thinking that if he didn't turn up at home or at work for a few days everyone might start thinking the worst. The only problem was that he couldn't get in touch with anyone because he didn't have a radio or anything with him. So he went down to the State Forestry Camp where there was a communications unit. The only trouble was that when he got there, the place was all shut up. So, with no one about, he thought they wouldn't mind if he broke into the State Forestry building, just to get the message through, like. So he did that. He broke in and got on the two-way radio.

As it turned out, the only people he could get hold of was the Royal Flying Doctor Service. So he explained things to the woman there and asked if she wouldn't mind giving his wife a ring, just to let her know that he was stuck in the forest and wouldn't be able to get home for three or four days. The woman who took the message at the Flying Doctor base said that that was fine and, when she'd finished talking to my brother-in-law, she called my sister.

'This is the Flying Doctor Service here,' she said. 'Your husband's just been in touch and he wanted us to let you know that he won't be able to get home for a few days because he's been rained in, up in the forest.'

As I said, around this particular time my sister and

my brother-in-law weren't seeing eye to eye and, what's more, he'd been spending a lot of time out on the town drinking and carrying on. So my sister thought that this was just another one of her husband's elaborate excuses and he'd talked some floozy of a barmaid into ringing through with the message.

Anyway, when the woman from the Flying Doctor Service had finished explaining my brother-in-law's situation, my sister replied in a very curt fashion, 'Oh, yes, and tell me, dear, just what hotel are you calling from?'

Fingers Off

There were only about sixty people living in Coober Pedy back when my pilot, Vic, and I flew there in the little Dragon DH 84. The main reason for that was they had no water. They didn't have water over in Andamooka either. Dry old places they were, and pretty wild too, I might add.

I remember the first time we went to Coober Pedy I did thirty-two tooth extractions in the one day. Bloody hard they were too. Some of those people out that way were as tough as nails. You'd have to be, just to live there. I tell you, I had a hell of a bad case of wrist drop the following day. Mind you, there wasn't even a proper dental chair. In those days all the tooth-pulling and so forth was carried out on a wooden box or a kitchen chair.

Then, after this day of tooth-pulling, Vic and I were getting ready to fly out to Andamooka and there was this chap who was an opal buyer at Coober Pedy. He's dead now. Funny bugger he was. A big chap. Anyhow, he asked if he could come along to Andamooka with us. The only problem that I could see was that we had an Aboriginal chap on board who had open TB, infectious TB. So I explained the situation to the opal buyer and he was still willing to come along.

'Yeah, that's all right by me,' he said.

Then I looked at Vic. 'Oh, yeah, suppose so,' was Vic's response.

Our first port of call on the way to Andamooka was a place called Coward Springs which is near the foot of Lake Eyre. Now the population of Coward Springs was focused around the publican and the station master. But, as they say, wherever there's a station master there's sure to be a railway station and I wanted to get this chap with the TB organised on a train so that he could go down to a decent hospital and receive the right treatment.

The problem with landing the Dragon at Coward Springs was that the town didn't have a proper airstrip. So Vic flew over the place and, to his surprise, he saw what he reckoned was a nice stretch of black gravel, perfectly situated alongside the railway line. 'What luck,' Vic said. So he put the Dragon down. And, by put down, I mean put down. Once we hit the ground we came to a shuddering halt in about 18 inches of bulldust which had a thin layer of gravel on top.

Anyway, after I got the Aboriginal chap organised to go on the train, we wandered over to the pub for a couple of beers. It was a hot day. When we came back I said to Vic, 'Well, Vic any idea how we're going to get the Dragon out of this bulldust and up in the air?'

The only thing that Vic could come up with was to run the plane up and down the strip a few times in an attempt to blow as much of the bulldust out of the way with the propellers as he could. It seemed to be a reasonable idea to me even though it'd create a bit of a dust storm in town. But the publican and the station master were pretty used to dust storms, living in a place like Coward Springs. So we explained what we were going to do to the opal buyer and he seemed to be okay with it as well.

'Yeah, that's all right by me,' he said.

So all was set.

'Youse blokes get in the plane, anyway,' Vic said to the opal buyer and me. 'You never know, if we get up enough airspeed I might have a go at taking off.'

Now take-off speed in the Dragon was about 70 miles an hour. The old plane travelled at about 80 or 90 miles an hour flat out, I think. So we tore up and down the strip a couple of times and moved some of the bulldust. By that stage, the best Vic had got the plane up to was about 60 miles an hour. The opal buyer was sitting in front of me in one of the canvas seats. Then, on the next go, Vic got the plane up to about 65 miles an hour.

'There's a chance we might have a go at this,' he shouted, 'so youse blokes make sure that you're well strapped in, just in case.'

By this stage we'd been there kicking up the dust for almost an hour, using up valuable fuel, and the opal buyer was getting a bit toey. So Vic gave the old Dragon all he had, which still wasn't quite enough. The tail was up but, instead of hauling off and coming back to have another go at blowing more bulldust out of the way, Vic tried to pull the aeroplane off the ground.

I could see from where I was sitting that we were heading directly towards a creek with some low, dead bushes in it. The opal buyer by this time had gone white with fear. But I could guess what Vic was up to — just the other side of the creek there was a clay pan and his idea was to hurdle the creek and hit the clay pan where he could get the Dragon up to speed for a decent take-off.

At that point I was in contact with the radio operator back at the base, a chap called Frank Basden. There I was talking away to Frank through the small microphone radio. It was one of those radios where you had to press a button when you were talking. So I've got my finger on the button and I'm saying to Frank 'We're just taking off from Coward Springs, Frank. I'll call you when we're in the air' when all of a sudden up jumps this opal buyer, out of his seat.

That was the last thing we needed, especially as we were about to hurdle the bushes in the creek. See, the Dragon's a very light aircraft. It's only made out of wood, canvas and string and you have to have it very well balanced, particularly on take-off, or it'd upset everything, the pilot and all. So I grabbed the opal buyer by the shoulder and dragged him back down into his seat and didn't I give him a serve or two. 'Sit down, you stupid so-and-so,' I said, and then proceeded to call him all the names under the sun.

So that was fine. We got over the creek, hit the clay pan, picked up speed, went about 80 yards, got off the deck and up we went, into the sky. When we arrived in Andamooka we said cheerio to the opal buyer and I went about my business.

By the time we got back to base, the incident with the opal buyer was almost forgotten. Then a few weeks later I received a letter from the Post Master General's Department which was in charge of the Department of Civil Aviation in Adelaide. What'd apparently happened was that, while I was giving the opal buyer a mouthful, I still had my finger down on the button of the radio microphone. At that point in time the Department of Civil Aviation was monitoring our radio frequency and, boy, they certainly sent a very terse notice concerning my use of obscene language over the national radio network.

From Bad to Worse

It was a terrible day to start with, a December day, and over 40° even at that early stage of the morning. What's more, the feeling was that things weren't going to get much better because all the dogs had gone under shade and there was no way they looked like they were keen on moving. It was only us of the human kind that went about our business, preparing to face the day.

And face it we did. At 9.30 am the Mount Isa Royal Flying Doctor Service received an emergency radio call from a vehicle that was bogged in bulldust about 8 kilometres south of Prospect Station. 'Where the hell's that?' I hear you ask. Well, for those who are interested, Prospect Station is about 350 kilometres north-east of Mount Isa, 150 kilometres south of Normanton and 250 kilometres north-west of Julia Creek. In other words, it's out there in the middle of nowhere.

But back to the story: what had happened was an elderly lady was driving along with two young teenagers in a Holden station wagon and they'd left the road, gone into a creek and run smack-bang into a tree. The kids were okay but the woman had suffered head injuries. Apparently, the station wagon wasn't too badly off but, when the teenagers had attempted to reverse it out of the creek, the vehicle got bogged in the bulldust.

Now I don't know if you've been bogged in bulldust or not but I can tell you that it's worse than being bogged in mud. So, there they were, stuck up to the axles. They couldn't go forward. They couldn't go backwards. So they called for help.

On this type of flight we usually carry a Flight Nurse with us but on this occasion, with three people being stuck out there, it was decided that only the doctor and I should go along. So, with me being the pilot, I fired up the Beechcraft Queen Air and we headed out to Prospect Station which was about an hour and a half's flying time away.

When we reached our destination, we circled low over the homestead only to find that it'd been abandoned. The upshot of that was, if we landed at Prospect there'd be no one to drive us out to the accident scene. And as the doctor stated, 'There's no way that I'm going to carry a stretcher for eight kilometres. Not under these conditions. It could well be the end of us.'

Still, I did a couple of dummy runs over the airstrip just in case. It was littered with ant hills so Prospect Station was out of the question, anyway. Our next best option was Esmerelda Station which was about 30 or

40 kilometres east of Prospect. More to the point, it was further away from the accident scene but, with little choice, we flew on.

When we arrived at Esmerelda Station there didn't look like there was much life in the homestead either. Still, the airstrip was in a much better condition so I put the Queen Air down and we waited in the hope that someone would come out and pick us up. Which didn't happen. So we wandered through the low scrub and sweltering heat, up and over the maze of dirt tracks and hills until we finally came upon the homestead.

'Is anybody there?' we called.

Not a sound. Esmerelda homestead had also been deserted.

So there we were, about 50 kilometres from the accident scene, with no transport. What's more, because of all the scrub, there was no way we could have flown back and landed any nearer to the bogged vehicle. So we hunted through the homestead and the outbuildings and there we stumbled across an old Toyota Landcruiser.

Now it was obvious that the vehicle hadn't been used for some time. For starters, it was about thirty years old. It was covered in a thick coating of dust. It was rusted. The tyres were perished. But, to our surprise, the keys had been left in the ignition. So we gave it a go and after a bit of pushing and shoving and mucking about we managed to get the old Toyota started. The only problem was that we didn't have a clue how much fuel was in the vehicle because none of the gauges worked.

With no fuel tanks in sight, that left us with a big worry, a big worry indeed.

'Will we chance it or won't we?' was the sixty-four million dollar question.

'Well, we've come this far, and it is an emergency,' echoed the answer.

So we decided to give it a shot.

As I said, there was a maze of tracks around the place, all going off in different directions. No signs, of course. What's more, because of the terrain, hilly and low gidgee scrub, we couldn't see for any great distance to get a decent bearing. Anyway, we followed something that resembled a once well-used track and somehow we ended up out on the main dirt road. Don't ask me how. I wouldn't have a clue. But we did.

There we were, driving down the road, hoping to hell that the Toyota wouldn't run out of fuel, when we saw the two young teenagers walking towards us through the shimmering mirage. They'd seen our plane fly over and they'd decided to head in the direction of where they thought it'd landed. By that stage these kids had trekked about eight kilometres in the searing heat, and they were terribly dehydrated. Terribly dehydrated.

So we picked them up, got some water into them, then we drove them back to their bogged vehicle. By now, a good hour or so had passed since we'd headed out in the old Toyota. When we got there, the elderly woman wasn't the best. Being as large as she was didn't help much either. It certainly hadn't been her day. Along with the head injuries, she was now suffering from severe dehydration to boot.

Anyway, the doctor got stuck in and started to sort the woman out. So there I was hanging around with nothing better to do than mull over the accumulation of the day's disasters. And it got me thinking, which was a big mistake, but that's what happens when I've got nothing better to do. Now, it was obvious that siphoning the petrol out of the Holden station wagon and putting it in the Toyota wouldn't work because the car ran on petrol and the Toyota ran on diesel. So that was out. But what could I do to save the situation? And the more I racked my brain, the more I started to formulate the idea that, if I dug the car out of the bulldust, all our troubles would be over and we wouldn't have to worry about running out of fuel in the Toyota.

So I grabbed a shovel and started to dig the car out. Now that was one of the most stupid things that a bloke could attempt to do, especially in 40° plus heat. As I said, even the dogs back in Mount Isa had crawled under the shade so that the sun wouldn't fry their brains. There I was, digging the wheels out, when I started to go all woozy.

'Oops,' I mumbled, and down I went like a sack of potatoes.

Well, that certainly put the doctor into a spin. He now not only had a dehydrated woman with head injuries plus two dehydrated teenagers on his hands, he also had a pilot who'd collapsed from heatstroke. And, what's more, without a pilot he knew that he couldn't go anywhere. He was well and truly stuck. So the doctor then had to turn around and rehydrate me.

Anyway, to cut a long story short, when I was feeling a little better we bundled everyone into the Toyota, got it going again, then headed back to Esmerelda Station. Now that was no real problem. But finding the airstrip from the homestead proved to be a different matter. Not only did we have the worry of not knowing how much fuel was left in the Toyota, we were all suffering from heatstroke to varying degrees. The old woman, in particular, was feeling it something terrible. What's more, the thermometer was still rising rapidly and we seemed to have lost our way among the myriad of tracks.

Then I started thinking again, which, as I said, was the worst thing I could possibly do. But it just seemed that, along every step of the way, things had gone from bad to worse to worser, if there's such a word. And I must admit, it was at that particular point in time that I started to have very grave doubts about any of us getting out of there alive.

So there we were, driving aimlessly through the rugged terrain, when the Toyota spluttered over a rise. And there she was, the aeroplane, the Queen Air — my Queen Air — sitting on the airstrip, waiting patiently for us.

God, she was the most beautiful sight I've ever seen in my life.

Great Break, Aye!

The life of a Flying Doctor is certainly a pretty demanding affair, I can tell you. And if it isn't these days, it certainly was when my husband, Tony, was working in the far north of Western Australia.

After we'd been back in Derby for twelve months, I distinctly remember us sitting down and working out that Tony hadn't had a single day's break and, mind you, that included the weekends. While we were living there he was responsible for the routine hospital work, the surgery, the clinics, the lot. And, because the dramas had no time schedule, rarely a night went by when he wasn't called out of bed. What's more, apart from annual holidays, we could only recall him having three days off in the past three years.

'Enough is enough,' I said. 'For one, you need a break. For two, we both need a break to spend some quality time together.'

So we decided to pack up the three kids and spend a nice, relaxing weekend as far away from it all as possible. To that end, the place we chose was the Australian Inland Mission Hospital out at Fitzroy Crossing.

After Tony had organised things on the work front to cover for his absence, the day finally arrived. Early one Saturday morning we loaded the kids into the car and drove the 300 or so kilometres across to Fitzroy Crossing.

Finally, we arrived. And what a relief. A whole weekend together lay ahead. What's more, the girls from the Inland Mission were so excited to see us. They'd even gone to the trouble of planning a big barbecue for the Saturday evening and had invited a few of the station people to come along, especially to meet the doctor and his family.

Anyway, we were just settling into our accommodation when Halls Creek sent through an emergency radio call to the Derby Base, informing them that a seven-year-old kiddie had accidentally shot a six year old in the chest. Of course, the Derby Hospital was without its doctor/surgeon, wasn't it, and not being able to deal with such an extreme case on their own, they got in touch with Tony.

The next thing I knew, the Queen Air aircraft had been dispatched from Derby and was on its way to pick up Tony at Fitzroy Crossing and take him to Halls Creek — which duly happened. Then at Halls Creek they picked up the gunshot victim and flew the child back to Derby Hospital. Tony remained there in surgery for most of the Saturday afternoon and into the night until he was confident that the child was out of danger and was on the road to recovery.

'Bugger it,' he said, 'I'm still going to have this weekend away with the family.'

So he asked the Matron at the Derby Hospital if he could borrow her car for a couple of days. This she agreed to and, at nine o'clock that night, Tony left Derby and drove the 300 or so kilometres back to Fitzroy Crossing to be greeted by a dinner of cold remains from the barbecue that'd been held in his, absent, honour.

Anyway, we finally wandered off to bed sometime later that night or, more than likely, early the following morning. By that stage, Tony was so exhausted he had trouble getting to sleep. But, not to worry, this was our weekend away from it all and we could take it easy and sleep in.

At seven o'clock on Sunday morning, Wyndham Hospital contacted Derby Hospital, who in turn rang Tony to inform him there'd been a very bad car accident involving three teenagers. One person had been killed and two were badly injured, one of whom had sustained severe head injuries. Tony was needed to do surgery.

However, during the three-way phone link-up between Wyndham Hospital, Derby Hospital and Tony at Fitzroy Crossing, an electrical storm hit and contact between the two hospitals was lost. It couldn't have happened at a worse moment. I mean, there they were, right in the middle of discussing blood groups and trying to organise whatever equipment Tony might need so that the hospital staff could get everything ready for when he arrived in Wyndham.

Anyway, the plane left the Derby Base at nine o'clock that morning and picked Tony up at Fitzroy Crossing, for the second time. I think they had a theatre sister and an anaesthetist on board on that trip as well, but I'm not sure. Off they flew to Wyndham where Tony remained in surgery all that day and well into the evening.

Tony eventually stabilised one of the lads enough for him to be sent down to Perth for further treatment. But the patient with the severe head injuries was a different matter. There were real problems there and it was deemed too dangerous to evacuate him to Perth along with his mate. So Tony stayed in Wyndham for the next three days monitoring the lad and helping him through that critical post-op period.

And, all this time, there I was in Fitzroy Crossing with the three kids and two cars, our own and the one that Tony had borrowed from the Matron. Now, I don't know how they got the Matron's car back to Derby. All I can remember is muttering a million times over, 'Great break, aye!' as I drove our car back home, across that 300 or so kilometres of damn road.

Gwen's Legacy

My friend Gwen had to go down to Adelaide in the Flying Doctor aeroplane a few years back. And on her way down she saw these little teddy bears in the plane. They were dear things, about 14 or 15 inches tall, all hand-knitted, with embroidered eyes and noses, and all of that.

'Oh,' she said to the Nursing Sister, 'they're just so cute. What are they for?'

'Well,' the nurse explained, 'they're what we call trauma teddies. If a child gets upset we give them a teddy to keep and explain that the teddy's got the same injuries that they have.'

The Nursing Sister also happened to mention that the Royal Flying Doctor Service was in desperate need for people to make the trauma teddies, on a voluntary basis. So Gwen said, 'Right, you're on. As soon as I get back home, I'll go to the Probus Club and the Senior Citizens and the CWA (Country Women's Association) and I'll get people knitting.'

But, as it turned out, when Gwen got down to

Adelaide she was diagnosed with terminal cancer so, when she arrived back home, she came to me. 'Audrey,' she said, 'I've made this promise to the Flying Doctor Service that I can't fulfil.'

Then she asked if I could start the trauma teddies off in the Riverland, which I was pleased to do. I went to the various community groups and explained how Gwen wanted the trauma teddies to continue and I asked if anybody else could pick up the basket because I was too tied up with other things. So a lady from the Lutheran Church took it on. And she's done a great job because now lots of groups in the Riverland are knitting trauma teddies, getting them ready to go down to be labelled for the Flying Doctor Service and their support services.

Anyway, I just mentioned that story because, even though Gwen's been dead for about three years now, her original promise has been more than fulfilled and no doubt those trauma teddies have helped many children and will continue to do so for a long, long time to come.

Handcuffed

To my knowledge Dr Clive Fenton was one of the rare 'true' flying doctors in as much as he was both an accomplished pilot as well as being a very good, and greatly admired, doctor. And when I say 'an accomplished pilot' I say that with a touch of mirth, as my story will reveal, because while Clive was a bit of a character, a real larrikin so to speak, he was also quite naughty at times, the daredevil type. Still, he did a tremendous amount of good up in the Northern Territory which was probably why he was able to get away with so much.

When I first ran into Clive, which was immediately after the war, Darwin was still under military control. And in those days, my late husband, Fred, an ex-RAAF Squadron Leader, had been appointed as the Regional Director of Civil Aviation. This was a posting that made him instrumental in assisting in the re-establishment of overseas air services, both in and out of Australia.

Anyhow, Clive and Fred didn't see eye to eye on

many issues. For starters, Clive didn't have too much respect for public servants. His favourite description of their livelihood was that of a 'dog-eat-dog' existence. So, when the new Department of Civil Aviation went about restructuring air traffic control, Clive dug his heels in. Though he still kept on flying, he steadfastly refused to obtain the appropriate pilot's licence.

It was then that the Department of Civil Aviation sent a directive, via my husband, insisting that Clive obtain this certain category of licence in accordance with the type of planes he was flying. Of course, Clive, being Clive, was of the mind that having already been a pilot during the war a licence issued by the DCA wasn't worth a fig.

'A complete load of administrative rubbish' was how he described the situation.

So dear old Clive completely disregarded the directive and continued on his unflappable way. Naturally, this type of behaviour riled the DCA. Yet they were caught between the devil and the deep blue sea because the only pilots who they could legally stop from flying were the ones who had been licensed under their own organisation and, of course, Clive had refused to get that particular licence.

Now a lot of people admired Clive for this particular stance. They saw him as someone who wasn't afraid to buck the system, a kind of Wild West maverick, a rough diamond.

But the DCA didn't see it that way. Yes, Clive was a delightful fellow and he was a proven pilot. No one could argue with that, what with his war record and all, but things were changing in Darwin. With so many people coming into Australia so soon after the war, the authorities just couldn't have these self-willed pilots out there doing their own thing.

For example, imagine the turmoil it might cause if a Constellation came into land and there was Clive doing a couple of loop-d-loops around the airstrip, which, I might add, was something that he'd been known to do. Another of his tricks was to put the wind up everyone by flying low over the open-air picture show at night or over people who were having a quiet picnic on the beach.

Now this might have been a great lark for Clive, but the DCA demanded order in the skies. So the Melbourne Headquarters became increasingly impatient with Clive and they said to Fred, 'You've got to get him licensed.'

So Fred followed it up and this is where my story comes in.

One evening everyone was gathered in the Darwin Club and the big talk of the moment was how Clive had refused, yet again, to get his licence. There they all were, Clive included. Now Clive liked a few drinks and after a while he saw Fred talking to the local sergeant of police. 'Watch this,' he said to his group of mates and he came over to Fred and the sergeant.

'Righto,' Clive said, holding out his hands. 'Here I am, you might as well handcuff me now and drag me off to prison.'

Then, as was usual with Clive, he put on a big song and dance about the whole affair. Anyway, this skylarking about started to get up the nose of the sergeant and he said to Fred, 'I'll fix him.' Quick as a flash the police officer took out his handcuffs and snapped them on Clive's wrists.

Well, this was a great joke, especially to Clive. He started wandering about the club, holding his glass in his handcuffed hands, amid much laughter and carry-on.

'Look what they've done to me,' Clive announced to all and sundry. 'They've finally arrested me.'

Oh, it was a real talking point.

Anyway, as the story goes, the sergeant got sick of all this carry-on and went home. So when Clive had had enough of the handcuffs and couldn't find the sergeant, he came over to Fred. 'Righto, Fred,' he said, 'the joke's over. You can take these things off now.'

'Sorry, Clive, no can do,' Fred said. 'The sergeant's gone home and he's taken the keys with him.'

'But you can't leave me like this,' Clive retorted.

Now Fred wasn't beyond having a bit of a joke himself. So he said to Clive, 'Well, Clive, the only thing that I can suggest is I take you down to the police station and you can wait there until the sergeant comes back on duty.'

'When'll that be?' asked Clive.

'I think he's gone to Alice Springs for a couple of days,' Fred said in a matter-of-fact way.

Well, Fred reckoned that you should've seen the look on Clive Fenton's face. The wind had really been taken out of his sails at that comment.

Heaven

I was stationed in Derby, living by myself at the time. There I was, a guy in his twenties with no commitments at all.

My wife-to-be was a community nursing sister over in Wyndham, and every week she drove down to the stations around the Halls Creek area, giving immunisations and that type of thing. Then every second Thursday, in order to link in with her previous clinic trips, I flew up there to pick up her and a doctor, and we did the follow-up air trips.

The standard procedure on those mornings was to get out of bed at about three o'clock. It'd be as black as the insides of a pig. I'd have a cup of tea, then drive to the airport, open up the hangar, push the Queen Air out, put the car in the hangar, and close the doors. Then I'd climb into this aeroplane, an aeroplane mind you, that someone had just about given me free rein to fly. It was virtually mine. And I'd fire this monster up, stoke up all the radios, call up on the HF frequency and talk to Perth or Port Hedland, whichever one was on duty.

'Perth (Port Headland), this is Foxtrot, Delta Victor, taxiing, Derby for Wyndham.'

And they'd come back sounding surprised, as they always did, thinking 'Who in their right mind would get out of bed at bloody three o'clock in the morning to go flying?'

Me.

So I'd taxi out, do all my run-ups and cockpit checks, then thunder down the runway, focusing on the instruments. As soon as I left the runway lights it was pitch black. Apart from the faint reflective light inside the windscreen, it was just a puddle of ink outside. Under those conditions there's no horizon. No visual reference. No bugger-all. I'd just focus on and fly the instruments.

Up I'd go. I'd turn left and climb towards 7500 feet. When I hit 7000 feet I'd engage the auto-pilot. Then I could relax. I was free.

There I was in this magnificent aeroplane at four o'clock in the morning, nobody within a million miles of me for all it mattered. And I'd sit back and look out the window at billions and billions and billions of stars. Each and every one of them was mine. I was in heaven, and heading to Wyndham for the six o'clock pick-up of the doctor and the nursing sister.

Kicking the Dust

Well, it's all just been pretty predictable stuff really. The evacuations that we've had to make out of here have gone off pretty much without a hitch. By 'here' I'm meaning Mount Vernon Station which is north of Meekatharra, in the central east of Western Australia.

Anyway, it's always amazed me how the Flying Doctor has been able to get in and out in quick-smart time. They're pretty efficient, you know, the lot of them — the doctors, the nurses, the pilots. We haven't even had any high-flaunting dramas about aeroplanes getting bogged in the bulldust or the mud like they have at other places. Still and all, there was one time I remember when the Flying Doctor plane was delayed from leaving our place, and that was for a bit of an odd sort of reason really, so I'll tell you about that one if you like.

As I said, the Flying Doctor plane has been able to get in and out in no time at all apart from this occasion when a young lad, a jackaroo he was, came off his horse and got his foot caught in the stirrup. Gee, he was in a mess. The poor kid had been dragged along the ground for a fair way and, among all that, the horse had trampled over him. I tell you, he was a pretty bruised and battered young man.

Anyway, we sent out an emergency for the Flying Doctor. When the plane arrived, on board was a doctor, a pilot and a nursing sister. So they settled the young stockman down and had just loaded him onto the plane when the nursing sister decided that she'd better go to the toilet before they flew back to the Meekatharra base.

'Sure,' I said and directed her off to the nearest loo, an outside construction it was. 'You go down this way and that, and it's just around the corner, over there, in that direction.'

Now one of the peculiarities of this particular toilet was that it had a metal door. So, when the sun shone on it, the metal expanded. Of course, we knew this and whenever we used the toilet we kept the door slightly open. But the nursing sister didn't, and with all the kerfuffle over the young stockman it completely slipped my mind to tell her. To make matters worse, this was a warm day, a very warm day indeed.

So off she went and the doctor completed what was necessary for the young stockman while the pilot did his pre-take-off checks. Some time passed and the nursing sister still hadn't returned. So there we were, standing around, trying to fill in the time with idle chat. And we waited and we waited until eventually we'd just about exhausted every avenue of conversation from the price of beef right through to the current climatic conditions . . . and still she hadn't appeared.

By this stage, the patient was looking quite distressed, the poor kid. What's more, the doctor seemed pretty anxious and the pilot was gazing at his watch then up at the skies then back at his watch again. So there we were, hovering around the plane kicking the dust with our boots, trying to think of what to talk about next, which we couldn't because all the while we were wondering what the hell was going on with the nursing sister.

Anyway, all this tension proved too much for my husband. 'Oh gee,' he blurted, 'I don't know, perhaps she isn't feeling too well.'

With this comment, the men turned to me. Being a female I put two and two together and came up with the obvious — that they weren't too comfortable about knocking on a toilet door to find out what a woman's problem might be.

'I'd better go and check on her, then,' I said.

'Good idea,' they chorused.

So I went over to the toilet and tapped on the door. 'Excuse me,' I said, 'but are you okay in there?'

'I'm in big trouble,' came the plaintive reply.

'What's up?' I asked, thinking the worst.

'The door's stuck and I can't get out.'

So I had a go at opening the thing and it was stuck, all right, stuck good and proper. What's more, it wouldn't budge no matter how hard I tried. Then I had to call the men around to have a go. God it was funny. If you can imagine the scene. There we were out in the middle of nowhere with these three men huffing and puffing and pushing and pulling at the door of the toilet which in turn was causing the complete structure to sway back and forward, and there was this poor woman stuck inside thinking that all her nightmares had come at once.

But they eventually managed to free it.

'One, two, three,' they called and gave an almighty pull.

The toilet door flung open and out stepped one very embarrassed nursing sister — as red as a beetroot, she was.

'Well,' she snapped, 'shall we go then?' And she strode off in the direction of the plane.

Knickers

I first became aware of the Royal Flying Doctor Service through a chap called Dr Clive Fenton. That was back during the war, like, when Clive was the Commanding Officer of No 6 Communications Unit, out at Batchelor, which was about 60 miles south of Darwin.

At that time, Clive was working solely as a pilot, not as a doctor. What's more, he had an excellent reputation as a pilot, one which was only surpassed by his dubious reputation of being a bit of a rouge, especially where the establishment was concerned. Clive simply refused to obey their rules. In actual fact he didn't obey much at all. He was pretty much a law unto his own. Still and all, I must say that, in my experience, I found him to be an extremely likeable and fair Commanding Officer.

But as well as being a pilot and a rogue and, no doubt, a good medical man, Clive was also a well-versed storyteller.

There's one story that sticks out in my mind, just for

starters. This incident happened when he was a Flying Doctor, back before the war. It involved either a Tiger Moth or a Fox Moth, I can't remember exactly. But it doesn't matter because both aircraft were two-seaters. Now what I mean by the planes being two-seaters is that, in both the Tiger Moth and the Fox Moth, the pilot sat in the back seat and the passenger sat directly in front of him, in the front seat. And to make matters more difficult there was no direct means of communication between one and the other.

Anyway, one day, Clive got a message to go out to pick up Mrs So-and-so from some station property. Miles away, it was. This Mrs So-and-so was due to have a baby and they were keen to get her into the maternity ward so that they could keep an eye on things. So Clive jumped into his plane and off he flew. But when he arrived, he checked this woman over and came to the conclusion that there was no real rush over the matter. In his medical opinion, she had another week or, perhaps, even two weeks up her sleeve.

But to save himself another long trip out to the property and back, Clive decided to take the woman back into the hospital anyway. So he positioned her in the front seat. He made sure that she was comfortable, then double-checked that she was okay. 'Are you sure that you're okay?' he asked. 'Yes,' she replied. Then he took off to return to the base. They'd been in the air for about half an hour when Clive noticed that the woman seemed to be in some sort of discomfort.

'She can't be,' he muttered to himself.

But the further on they flew, the more this woman's discomfort seemed to increase, and before long, there she was, twisting this way and that. Now the more that this woman wriggled about, the more Clive began thinking that his previous diagnosis might've been a week or two off the mark. It'd happened to doctors before. You couldn't always be right. Nothing's 100 per cent certain. Perhaps the stress and vibration of the flight was bringing the baby on prematurely. But it was only when the situation reached desperation point and the woman attempted to lift herself out of the seat that Clive's concern turned to panic.

'Hell,' he said, 'the baby's coming.'

So Clive was left with no other option than to put the plane down, and put it down mighty quick, or there could be big trouble. Now it isn't the easiest thing in the world to put a plane down in the middle of nowhere, especially when that 'middle of nowhere' happens to be nothing but desert and scrub. So he searched around the area and the first piece of half reasonable land he came across, he took the bit between the teeth and went for it.

Now, as you might well imagine, landing a plane in those sorts of geographical conditions was a precarious exercise at the best of times. But with a woman on board who was on the verge of giving birth, Clive was fully aware that any sudden bumps or violent shaking may well get the birthing process rolling before he could attend to the situation.

But as luck and good flying skills would have it,

Clive managed to make a reasonably smooth landing. Then as soon as the plane came to a halt he shouted, 'Keep calm. Keep calm. Breathe nice and deep. First, I'll get you out of the plane and we can take things from there.'

Then he grabbed his medical bag, jumped out and raced around to tend to the woman. It was at that point that Clive happened to notice a strange, sheepish look on the woman's face. Now this particular facial expression caused him to do a double take.

'You are about to have the baby, aren't you?' he said.

'No,' whispered the woman.

'Then why all the discomfort in the passenger's seat?' he asked.

'Me undies got all knotted up,' she replied.

Love is . . .

Remember back in the 1970s when they had those little logos — 'Love is . . . something-or-other'? For example, 'Love is . . . not having to say you're sorry'. Well, there's a saying around here that goes 'Love is . . . not pressing charges', and that stems from the time when we had an emergency flight to a town where there'd been a domestic dispute.

What had happened was that this fellow and his de facto wife had come home after a session on the grog, they'd had a blue and, amongst the turmoil, she'd picked up a large kitchen knife and knifed him in the chest. Down he went like a sack of potatoes with the knife sticking out of him and blood gushing everywhere. When the woman realised what she'd done, she panicked, rang the ambulance, and before they arrived she nicked off out bush.

As you might imagine, it was quite a mess and the victim wasn't in the best of conditions. That's when we got the call to fly out and pick him up.

Anyway, they brought this fellow out to the airport

so that we could load him straight onto the plane. There were a couple of policemen in tow, just in case. At that point the fellow was conscious and still had the large kitchen knife embedded in his chest. Then, as we started to wheel him out to the plane, his de facto appeared out of nowhere. She'd seen us come in to land, realised what was going on, and had rushed out to the airport. But just as she started to run towards the plane, she was grabbed by the two police officers.

If you can imagine the scene, there we are, loading this critically injured fellow onto the plane. And there's this woman being restrained by two policemen. And with the tears flowing down her face, she starts sobbing out at the top of her voice, 'I'm sorry, darlin'. I didn't mean ta do it!'

And this fellow, there he is with the knife sticking out of his chest. Well, he struggles to raise himself and he starts calling back at the woman, 'That's all right, sweetheart. I forgive yer!'

Then she replies, 'I love yer, darlin', honest I do!'

'I love yer too,' the fellow calls out. 'And don't worry about a thing, sweetheart,' he says, 'I'm not pressing charges!'

Mayday! Mayday!

It was, um, October 19th, actually. I was about nine months pregnant at the time and still working in Derby as a Flight Nursing Sister. Not that there was much flying for me. I'd been thrown off the aeroplane because I was bigger than most by that stage with my bub being due fairly soon. Anyway, my husband, Jan, had gone off flying the aeroplane, doing a clinic circuit with a doctor and a nurse, and I was back at the base doing a radio session.

You know about the radio sessions, don't you? Well, I used to go on air and ask if anybody wanted drugs or medications for their station's medical chest and, if so, I'd organise for them to be sent out. Also, sometimes people just wanted to ask general questions about health and so forth so that they wouldn't make idiots of themselves when the doctor came on line. In other words, I did a lot of trouble shooting.

So there I was chatting on to people and I got the strong feeling that Jan was listening in from the aeroplane because he often used to count the times that I said 'um' over the radio. As you might have gathered, um, it's a little habit of mine, though I'm getting better. Anyway, Jan used to count my 'ums' and he'd give me a bit of backchat. It was just a fun thing, really.

So I'd just finished my part over the radio and the doctor came in and sat down and said, 'Good morning. And what're the stations for medicals today?'

Just at that point, Jan came over the radio. 'Mayday! Mayday!' he called.

'Oh, shit,' I blurted out, because I'm sort of a vocal person.

'What on earth did he say?' the doctor asked.

'Mayday,' I said. Then I asked Jan, 'What's your problem?'

'My wing's on fire,' came the reply.

Apparently, Jan had left Tableland Station with the doctor, the nurse and some patients on board, and they were heading down to Lansdowne Station, in the north-east of Western Australia. So there he was, flying along at about 3500 feet when he looked out the window and the whole top of the left wing was going black and buckling. What's more, the aeroplane was trailing a plume of black oily smoke.

That's when he called through with the mayday.

'Okay, Jan. That's okay,' I kept saying as he explained the situation and gave his location, in case they went down. When he'd finished giving me the details, he said, 'I'm going to the other frequency. Over and out.'

'Okay,' I said, 'anything else I can do?'

'No,' he replied and radio contact ceased.

Just then, one of our doctors who'd overheard our conversation came rushing in and said, 'What's he done to my aeroplane?'

'Oh, he's just had a bit of an accident,' I replied, in a manner that came over as, perhaps, far too casual.

Now my being so calm took everyone aback because they imagined the instant panic that they'd go into if they knew that it was their spouse stuck up there, at 3500 feet, in an aeroplane that was on fire.

But it didn't happen to me. Even though I knew that things must've reached an extremely critical stage for Jan to have put through the mayday call, it was almost like I had a premonition that everything was going to be okay. There was nothing to worry about. Jan was in control. Jan would save the day.

Much to everyone's complete amazement, after Jan had gone off air I carried on with our medical schedules, 'scheds' as they're called. And the doctor carried on with me. So I just kept right on going and finished off the scheds, and when they were done we went back to find out what Jan was up to.

As it turned out, after the mayday call, Jan had shut the left engine down in case it was contributing to the problem. But unbeknown to him at the time, the fuel tank had ruptured in the left wing and the wiring loom had set fire to it. So not only was the wing on fire but by that stage it'd burnt the flap controls out, leaving him with full flap condition on one side and none on the other. It's called an asymmetric flap condition.

Then after he shut the engine down, he dropped the landing gear in case the fire raged through into the undercarriage as well. By that time things were starting to get pretty interesting from a flying point of view. But Jan being Jan, he somehow managed to wrestle the burning aeroplane onto the ground at Lansdowne Station. When it rolled to a stop he got everybody outside to safety. With that done he went back and grabbed the fire extinguisher from inside and managed to put the fire out.

So, my premonition had been right, after all. Jan had, um, saved the, um, day, thankfully.

Missing

During 1955–56 I was working on Troughton Island which is just off the far north coast of Western Australia, out in the Timor Sea. The island itself was quite small, only about three-quarters of a mile long and half a mile wide. A year and a bit I was there, employed at a government high-frequency direction-finding station, keeping track of shipping movements in the area.

In early February '56, I got a toothache; pretty bad it was, so we flagged down a passing ship which took me to the mainland, to Wyndham in fact. There I went to see the local doctor in the hopes that he'd be able to extract the tooth.

'Not my cup o' tea,' he reckoned.

This doctor was an Australian Rugby Union international. As strong as a bull, he was. But when it came to pulling teeth, especially without the aid of anaesthetic, he went to water.

'Well, you've got to have a go,' I said. 'The pain's killing me.'

So he did.

But no matter how hard he tried, he couldn't remove the tooth. As a last resort, he suggested that we go down to the local drinking establishment and have a few whiskies. The object there was to induce an anaesthetic effect on me and for him to gain some much needed Dutch courage. So we did that, and when we came back he had another go at the tooth. That didn't work either so we headed off down to the local watering hole again for a top-up.

We did this a few times, back and forward, back and forward, but still the tooth wouldn't budge. By this time neither of us could walk a straight line.

'Best I can do is to get yer to Darwin,' he slurred, and added that there was a plane passing through in a couple of days.

So I cadged a lift on that plane. Bugger of a trip it was, with the thing landing at every station and halfway house between Wyndham and Darwin, dropping off grog and supplies. Mostly grog, I might add. It was pretty wild out there in those days. And on every landing, the station people were sympathetic to my problem and plied me with a top-up of 'anaesthetic'.

By the time we landed at Darwin airport I was anaesthetised to every inch of my body, except where it mattered — to the aching tooth. My cheek had puffed up like a balloon. When I finally saw the dentist he took one look, put his hand in my mouth, gave the tooth the gentlest of tweaks and . . . out it came, just like magic.

It was while I was in Darwin that the Flying Doctor Service over in Derby got a call from an outlying property. The station manager's baby was very sick so they flew out there. The weather was atrocious. Anyway, they arrived safely at the station, picked up the sick child and the mother, and took off again to return to base.

On their way back, they went missing.

A search was mounted and a plane with direction-finding equipment on board was flown from Perth up to Darwin. Somehow the news had spread that I was in town so they contacted me to go out in a search aircraft. My job was to pick up the automatic distress signal which the pilot would've set off the moment that he knew he was in strife. If we heard the signal then we could pinpoint where the plane was and go in and get the survivors. To help us in our mission all transmitting stations throughout Australia which ran on that particular frequency were shut down for an hour or so.

So we set off and flew over the search area. Extremely rugged country it was. Up and down we went, this way and that. But I never heard a sound.

Then later that month, the wreckage of the plane was discovered in the King Leopold Ranges, out from Derby. They'd flown straight into a cliff face. All five people on board had been killed.

Mission Impossible

They say that you can't do the impossible. And I'd have to go along with that. If something's impossible to do, then it's impossible to do it. You can't do it. It's impossible. Full stop. But I'll give you a tongue twister. I reckon that the Flying Doctor Service has gone as close to doing the impossible as it's possible to do, and on quite a few occasions, too, I might add.

Why, just a year or so ago there was this young geophysicist chap. He and his survey crew were correcting boundaries by satellite, out in the Tirara Desert, beyond the Simpson Desert, in probably one of the most isolated parts of Australia.

One morning, around 8 o'clock, this young chap left the camp to go out and do some survey work. There he was in his Landrover, driving through the bush, when he came upon a desert taipan. Now these things are the most venomous snakes in Australia, even more so than the Cape York taipan, and they're pretty deadly. So what he did was he ran over this blinking five-foot-long snake. The trouble was that he made a slight error of judgment and ran over the tail section of the snake and not the body as he'd intended.

He must have had his elbow resting out the window at the time because this snake bounded up like lightning... Zap... and latched onto him. There he was driving along with the fangs of this desert taipan embedded in his arm. The more he tried to shake the thing off the tighter it latched on, and the tighter it latched on the more poison it pumped into him. Eventually, he shook the snake off and he got on his Traeger radio and called up his camp.

'I've just been bitten by a hell of a snake,' he exclaimed.

'Well, you'd better get back here quick and we'll start to get things happening at this end,' his mate replied.

So his mate called the Flying Doctor Service in Broken Hill.

'What sort of snake's he been bitten by?' the doctor asked.

Now that was something no one knew at the time, not even the lad, but to be on the safe side the doctor said that they'd fly up there immediately and bring along as many vials of antivenene as he could find. So, after they sorted out where the nearest airstrip was, the mate got onto Santos in the Moomba gasfields who said they'd send up a helicopter, post haste, to transport the lad from the camp to the airstrip.

So the Flying Doctor plane, a Super King Air, arrived at the designated outback airstrip, a map reference of about 30 miles from where the boys were camped. Not long after, the helicopter arrived with the young chap aboard. By this stage the lad was almost unconscious. It was touch and go so the doctor pumped some antivenene into him. Then they whipped him into the aircraft where the doctor gave him another shot which he apparently had a severe reaction to.

They took off from this dirt airstrip which was, as I said, out in one of the most remote parts of Australia, and in just under an hour they had the young fellow in intensive care in the Royal Adelaide Hospital.

Now that's as close to achieving the impossible as you can get, I reckon. What's more, the lad lived and is now back on the job. He should have died but he didn't. It was just one of those miracles of survival, one that even surprised the young chap. When he woke up two days later, the first thing he said was, 'Tell Mum I'm still alive!'

Mud Happens

Just the day to go out wearing my new Rossi boots instead of my normal old nurse's shoes. Just the day to wear a good pair of pants instead of shorts. But it was cold, and we were heading out to a cattle station just north of Alice Springs where I knew that it'd be much colder.

An old station owner had been driving along in the manner that old farmers do when his ute hit a bump. Up he went and when he came down again, he smashed his chest on the steering wheel.

'He might'a cracked some ribs, I reckon,' a young jackaroo had told us over the radio.

It'd been raining so we asked the jackaroo if he knew what condition the airstrip was in. 'Just hang on a tick,' he said. There was some shouting in the background before the jackaroo came back on. 'The old bloke says yer won't have any trouble at all,' he said. 'Reckons it's as good as gold, as good as gold.'

Still, the pilot waited for a strip report to confirm that it was okay and then off we went, out to pick up this old man, just the pilot and myself. There wasn't a doctor on that trip. There was no real need, really. It was a simple evacuation. In and out, and back to Alice Springs.

The clouds were quite heavy so we stayed low. Then when we arrived, the pilot flew over the runway just to double-check its condition. Everything seemed okay, just like the old bloke had said, 'as good as gold'. The young jackaroo was down there waiting with the man. A young jillaroo was also there. So we landed and loaded the old boy onto the plane. About eighty he was. As deaf as a post. A cantankerous old bugger to boot.

'What're yer doin'?' he asked.

'I'm checking your blood pressure,' I said.

'Me what?'

'Your blood pressure,' I shouted.

Everything was 'What's that?' or 'What're yer doing?' Then I'd have to repeat myself before he understood. It was just that he didn't hear properly.

Anyway, it was about 10.30 in the morning when we got the old bugger settled in the plane. We said goodbye to the young jackaroo and the jillaroo, who turned out to be brother and sister. Over from Queensland they were. One had been there a week, the other for about three months.

So the pilot taxied to the end of the strip to prepare for take-off, which was the end from where we'd landed. As he was sweeping the plane around in a wide arc, we came to an abrupt halt. There was this sinking feeling, and down we went into a well-disguised, grassy bog.

Now, bogging an aeroplane is one of the worst things that can happen to a pilot. It's something they're never likely to live down, a stigma that stays with them for the remainder of their days. And our pilot was well aware of the fact. But what made it all the more painful in this case was that he'd been given a strip report that assured him everything was okay. So, there he was, up the front, slapping the dashboard and swearing to the heavens.

So I let the pilot be. When he'd settled down we got out and inspected the situation. It didn't look good. We were in deep. Mud was halfway up the front wheel and also the right-hand side wheel.

'What's wrong?' the old farmer called from inside the plane.

'We're bogged,' I shouted.

'We're what?'

'We're bogged!'

'Could've told you it were soft up this end.'

The pilot and I raised our eyebrows to the heavens and, without saying a word, we agreed to leave the old chap inside while we had a go at lifting the plane out of the bog. So, with the two young kids helping us, we pushed. We pulled. We shoved. We dragged. But the plane wouldn't budge. So I opened the door of the aircraft to see how the old bloke was going.

'What's goin' on out there?' came a familiar voice.

'We're still bogged,' I called back.

While the brother and sister went back to the homestead to get another four-wheel-drive vehicle, the pilot called our mechanics in Alice Springs to find out where to tie the towropes so that the undercarriage wouldn't get damaged as we were pulling the plane out. Then the kids arrived back, loaded to the hilt with more towropes, bog-mesh, shovels, fence posts and chains. So we dug around the wheels, hooked up the towropes to the four-wheel drives and we pulled. 'Snap' went the towropes.

'Bugger,' I said, then looked down at my mud-soaked Rossi boots and long pants. 'Double bugger.'

But we didn't give up. We dug out more mud, retied the towropes, laid down the bog-mesh, hooked up the vehicles and pulled again. This time — 'Whoosh' — the wheels went straight through the bog-mesh and deeper into the mud. So we dug some more, then tried putting chains under the wheels for traction. That didn't work either. It seemed like nothing was going to work.

For a fleeting moment we even considered sitting the old bugger outside on a chair and getting him to help out with a few directions and suggestions. But that was for only a fleeting moment.

'Used ta be a swamp down this end, it did,' he shouted, 'but we filled it in ta' make the airstrip.'

'I thought you said it was as good as gold,' I said.

'What?' he called.

'I said, I thought that you told us that the strip was as good as gold!'

So we dug some more and we tried packing timber around the wheels, and still the plane wouldn't budge. By this stage the pilot was about ready to give up.

'Come on,' I said, 'just a little bit longer, just keep trying.'

The other option was to borrow the front-end loader from Utopia, an Aboriginal community about 30 kilometres away. Utopia, by the way, is the place where Aboriginal dot painting first began. But, from where we were, Utopia was a good hour or so's drive, over and back, which would've meant that we'd have to stay the night out there in the company of you-know-who.

So, desperate measures had to be taken. And they were. I straddled the cockpit and opened the window so that I could hear, then I tried to steer with my feet in an attempt to keep the nose wheel straight. But that didn't work either. So we grabbed some metal fence posts, 'star-droppers' they're called, and we laid them sideways under the wheels in the hope they might act like a little ramp. And it worked, and we finally managed to pull the plane out. Over four hours it'd taken. But we'd done it. We were out.

'What's goin' on now?'

'We're out of the bog.'

'We're what?'

'We're out of the bog!'

'Let's have a cup o' tea and some biscuits, then,' he said.

So we did. Apart from my wrecked Rossis and

pants, things could've been worse. We were just lucky that the cranky old bugger's injuries weren't more serious than they were. But the person who I really felt sorry for was the pilot. He knew he was going to be in for a hell of a ribbing when we got back to Alice Springs. And he was.

The moment we arrived, the engineers appeared on the scene. 'We weren't worried, Penny,' they said. 'We knew a country girl like you would get him out o' trouble.'

Night Eyes

One day we got a call from this chap who was up in the Flinders Ranges, in the north of South Australia. He said that he'd been following a car along a dirt road when it'd overturned, leaving two ladies stuck inside with bad injuries. A third woman, who was also hurt, had been able to free herself from the vehicle. When we asked the bloke his whereabouts, he gave his location as being near a certain airstrip in the national park.

'We'll meet you there, then,' we said.

'No worries,' he replied. 'I'll stay with the ladies until I see your plane coming in then I'll drive straight out and pick you up.'

'Okay,' we said, 'we'll be there ASAP.'

Now, attempting to land a plane in the Flinders Ranges is a difficult task at the best of times, especially in the national park. Firstly, it's quite mountainous in places and, secondly, the airstrips are extremely short. But the pilot was willing to give it a go just as long as we could get out of there before dark. Getting out before dark was the least of our problems. We had plenty of daylight hours up our sleeve. What's more, with the accident occurring near the airstrip as the bloke had said, things were set for a speedy evacuation.

So we flew to the airstrip that the chap had mentioned but when we landed no one came out to meet us. We waited for a while. Then we waited for a little while longer, and still he hadn't turned up. Eventually, we radioed through and found out that the chap had mistakenly given us the name of the wrong airstrip and the accident had occurred about 30 or 40 kilometres down the road.

'Here we are,' said the doctor, 'stuck in the middle of nowhere with no visible means of road transport and the accident victims are stuck in their car down the track' — which just about summed the situation up, really.

We were scratching our heads, considering our minimal options, when a cloud of dust came around the corner. And out of that cloud of dust appeared a small tourist bus. At the sight of the bus we ran over and blocked the road to make sure that it'd stop.

Now when the bus driver pulled up you'd swear that a couple of those tourists thought it was a hold-up because video recorders and cameras disappeared from view and their eyes glazed over with fear. I don't know what they were thinking. Maybe they thought that we were the Kelly gang in disguise or something and I was Ned Kelly in drag, all dressed up in a nurse's uniform for the occasion. I don't know. What's more, we didn't take the time to check. We were too busy telling our tale of woe to the driver and asking if he could drive us down to pick up the injured people.

'That's fine,' he said. 'Anything to be of help.'

Then he told the tourists that they had to get out of the bus, which was something that a few of them didn't look too keen on doing, I might add.

'No, no. No robbery,' he said, trying to allay their fears. 'No, no. No hijack. Everything fine-and-dandy.'

When the last of the tourists was evicted, we loaded our medical gear into the small bus and jumped aboard. Then the driver took off, leaving the pilot behind to attempt to explain to the tourists why they'd been dumped in the middle of the uninhabitable wilds of Australia, as they saw it.

When we arrived at the scene of the accident we finally met up with the bloke who'd given us the name of the wrong airstrip and together with the bus driver we all managed to get the two ladies out of the car. Once we'd stabilised them we placed them in the bus and started to head back to the airstrip.

Now, because of the extent of the injuries and the poor condition of the road we were only able to travel at a snail's pace and that left us in a very tricky situation. Along with all the other cock-ups during the day, the sun had already set and darkness was falling at a rate of knots. By the time we arrived back at the airstrip it was pitch black. But the pilot hadn't been hanging around idly discussing the pros and cons of bushranging to the tourists. Not on your life.

When we'd flown in, he'd noticed that the national parks people were doing some roadworks further down the track, and after we'd left he'd rounded up a couple of graders and a few other vehicles. So as we were loading the injured ladies onto the plane, they positioned the vehicles along each side of the airstrip, ready to turn their lights on so we could see where to take off. What's more, when they'd run out of vehicles they filled up all the tin cans they could find with kerosene or diesel and used them as flares to help light the strip.

Now that in itself was an amazing piece of resourcefulness but the rescue still relied on the pilot's ability to fly us out of there. As I said, it was quite mountainous, the airstrip was extremely short, and by this time it was pitch dark, around 9 or 10 pm. Then, as we were taxiing down the runway, another problem popped up. And when I say 'popped up', I mean popped up. With it being a national park, a million and one kangaroos appeared out of the bush to see what all the hoo-ha was about.

With the doctor in the back of the plane attending to the accident victims, I was up front alongside the pilot. As we picked up speed down the runway the noise of the engines spooked the kangaroos. In blind panic they started hopping all over the airstrip, left, right and centre.

I sat there, frozen with fright as the pilot threaded the plane through the startled kangaroos then made a sharp ascent up through the mountains and into the sky.

'Wow,' I gasped in astonishment at the pilot's skill. 'I must say that that was an amazing piece of flying.'

Then I heard his faltering voice ask, 'Is it safe to open my eyes now?'

No Thanks!

He was only a young lad, a jackaroo at Innamincka Station. Pretty new to the game he was. Anyway, he went into Innamincka and got stuck into the grog. Then on his way back out he came across a snake. Being young and stupid and, more to the point, pissed to the eyeballs, he tried to be smart and pick the thing up. The obvious happened — he got bitten. That's when we got the call.

'Look,' said the manager from Innamincka Station, 'I don't know how much of this is bullshit or not but we've got a kid here who's as drunk as a skunk and saying that he's just been bitten by a snake.'

We took the call like it was a life and death situation — which in actual fact it proved to be. An Inland Taipan it was, one of the most venomous snakes you're likely to find. Trouble being, time was against us. In cases like that, the sooner the initial treatment is carried out the better chance the patient has of survival. As it stood, it would have taken the Flying Doctor Service too long to fly from Broken Hill down to Innamincka then get a lift out to the station to give that treatment. So, with me being at Moomba, in the gasfields, Santos offered to helicopter me out there straight away to have a look at this kid.

It was a woeful night. The wind was blowing a gale by the time the pilot and I set off. Then just as the lights of Innamincka Station come into view, all hell broke loose. The helicopter suddenly went into free fall. It was like being at the top floor in a lift and the wires snapping. The air vanished from under us. The rotor blades were still whirling. There was nothing the pilot could do. Down we came from an awful height. Crunch! We hit the ground and bounced a couple of times before the helicopter flipped over on its top with the blades still spinning. There was screeching, groaning, sparks. Then they ground to a stop. Silence.

The pilot and I sat in our seats, upside down. It took a while to register that we were still alive.

'Are you all right?' the pilot finally asked.

'I think so,' I replied.

'Guess we'd better get out of here, then,' he said.

'Guess so,' I replied.

So he undid his safety belt and fell to the top of the bubble of the helicopter. I followed and down I came, right on top of him. Poor bloke. Cracked his ribs or something. I can't remember now. But, miraculously, they were the only injuries either of us received apart from general bruising and things.

As we were sorting ourselves out, the strong smell

of fuel started to fill the cab. I had visions of the helicopter exploding in a massive fireball like they do in those American movies. The pilot must have seen the same films. 'Let's get out of here,' he called, and we scampered from the wreckage and took to the bush.

Thankfully, the station manager had been waiting outside the homestead for us to arrive in the helicopter. He'd seen the lights come over the hill, then disappear. Thinking the worst he jumped into his ute and came looking for us. The pilot and I must have been running on adrenaline because the manager reckoned he found us about four kilometres from the upturned helicopter.

The odd thing was, though, when we arrived back at the homestead all those years of nurse's training took over. To this day I can't remember having one thought pass through my mind about how battered and bruised I was or just how close to death we'd come. My total focus was on the patient.

Things weren't looking too good for the lad, though. He'd passed out, which only clouded the issue. How much of his comatose state owed itself to drunkenness and how much to the snake bite was difficult to tell. I stabilised him the best I could and made sure that the Flying Doctor Service at Broken Hill were on their way down to pick him up. Then we drove the kid into Innamincka. With it being night, the locals came out to help light flares along the airstrip so that the plane could land. Trouble was, the strong winds kept blowing all the flares out.

Anyway the RFDS pilot circled a few times, summing up the situation. It was just too risky to attempt to land without flares to light up the strip and they decided to fly on to Moomba, hijack the ambulance, and come out and meet us halfway. So with the lad still out to it from the effects of the alcohol and the snake bite we headed off to meet them. Down the track a way the ambulance came into view. I can tell you, it was one of the most welcoming sights of my life.

'Thank God you're here,' I said.

So we stacked the lad into the ambulance and the doctor took over. The lad was taken back to Moomba then flown to Broken Hill. His life was saved. He recovered okay. The odd thing was, though, and I'm just not on about myself here, a lot of people put their lives at risk or volunteered their time and effort to save that lad, and not even one word of thanks. Never.

Off

It's not like being a normal doctor, working as we do, away out here. You haven't got the luxury of being able to sit down, face to face with a patient to make a learned diagnosis. What's more, more often than not the initial contact is carried out through a third party. So you have to be a bit of a mind reader as well as having a good grounding in the bush lingo.

Imagine, for example, a new doctor, fresh to the Flying Doctor Service with hardly any experience of bush people at all. Some bloke's taken ill, way out on a remote station somewhere. Normally, those types of males feel awkward about talking to a doctor about their problems, let alone anyone else, so the wife's the initial contact.

'Hello, doctor, me hubby's taken crook,' she might say.

'What do you mean, crook? How crook is he?' the doctor would ask.

'Darl, the doctor wants to know how crook yer are,' she says, asking her hubby.

'Tell him I'm as crook as a dog,' comes the chap's voice.

'Doctor, he reckons he's real crook.'

'Can you give me some idea as to where he's feeling crook?'

'Darl,' she asks, 'the doctor wants to know where yer feeling crook?'

'Christ, woman, I'm feeling crook all over.'

'Doctor,' she says, 'Hubby reckons he's feeling crook all over.'

'Well,' says the doctor, 'before I can prescribe treatment, we've got to isolate the problem area, okay? So let's start from the top. Is he crook in the head?'

'Darl, the doctor wants to know if yer crook in the head.'

'What sort o' bloody question's that?' echoes the gruff voice. 'Course I'm not bloody crook in the head, woman. I'm as sane as the next bloke. Sounds to me like he's the one who's crook in the head, not me.'

'No doctor, he's not crook in the head.'

'Well, is he crook in the abdomen?'

'In the what?' she asks.

'The abdomen. The stomach.'

'Oh, you mean the guts!' she says. 'Darl, are yer crook in the guts?'

'Too bloody right I'm crook in the guts! That's the bloody reason I'm calling the idiot.'

'Yes, doctor, he's crook in the guts.'

'Has he got nausea?'

'Nausea? What's nausea?'

'Has he been vomiting?' says the doctor.

'What?'

'Has he been spewing?'

'No, I don't think he's been spewing. Darl, yer haven't been spewing again, have yer? No doctor, he hasn't been spewing.'

'Well, has he opened his bowels today?'

'What do yer mean by "opened his bowels"?'

'Has he had a crap?'

'Darl, have yer done number two's yet, today?'

A loud call of 'No!' is heard in the background.

'No, doctor, he hasn't done one of those.'

'Well, has he voided?'

'What's that?'

'Has he urinated?'

'Urinated? What's that?' she asks.

'For God's sake, has he had a piss?'

'No need to get angry, doctor,' comes the reply. 'Darl, the doctor wants to know if yer done a number one today.'

'Tell him to mind his own bloody business!'

'He's not sure, doctor.'

And so the conversation continues until the doctor eventually eliminates the possibilities and hones in on the problem.

But sometimes, of course, it gets more serious than that, a lot more serious. Like the time we were doing a clinic out at Thargomindah and the emergency beacon was activated on the HF radio. A station fellow was calling from about three-quarters of an hour's flying time away, saying that there'd been an accident.

As it turned out, a motor cyclist was on his honeymoon and he'd been riding along with his wife in the side car. They'd come to the end of the bitumen section and hit the gravel. He'd lost control, veered off over the table drain, and his leg got caught between the motor bike and a mulga tree. His wife was okay but he wasn't. As I heard it over the radio, the station fellow said that the motor cyclist had his leg broken.

To piece the situation together, I began with a few questions. Firstly, how did he know the leg was broken, to which I received the sharp reply of 'Yer'd have to be blind not to see that it's broken, doc'. So that established that. Then I asked which leg was it, right leg or left leg. Was it broken above the knee or below the knee. 'Above the knee,' I was told. Then I asked if it was bleeding.

'Yes,' the station fellow said, 'it's bleeding quite badly.'

So I questioned him about the bleeding. Was it was seeping from the breakage point or was the blood spurting out.

'It's spurting out,' came the reply.

'How far?' I asked.

'Oh, only about four or five yards,' he said.

Well, that told me something. I imagined the situation again. A motor cyclist, still alive, thankfully, but in deep shock. The accident. The bike. The tree. A leg which had been broken. The spurting blood. It must surely have been a severed artery. That was the first problem we had to sort out. So, I told the station fellow to apply pressure to the bleeding spot and try to contain the bleeding.

So we activated the plane and off we flew. We were met at the airstrip in a ute and driven to the scene of the accident. It was only as we drove up to the motor cyclist that the whole story was revealed. The mental picture I'd drawn was complete, apart from one major discrepancy. The station fellow forgot to inform me of one very important fact about the broken leg. The leg wasn't just broken, it'd been broken completely ... off. And there was the motor cyclist, sitting under the tree, and propped up beside him was his severed leg.

Old Bill McDougall

Old Bill McDougall lived in a dilapidated caravan at White Dam, about 10 kilometres out of the small opal-mining town of Andamooka, in central South Australia. And alongside the caravan he built a tin shed which became widely known as, amongst other things, the 'Ettamogah Pub'. The reasoning behind that was, the place looked in worse condition than the cartoon of its namesake.

Anyway, Old Bill and his Ettamogah Pub gained quite a reputation. They became a tourist spot. People from all over used to go out there just to visit. And, as a lot of these travellers were going around Australia, they'd 'borrowed' road signs and the like to specially deliver to Old Bill. So signs like 'A new McDonald's restaurant is about to be built here' or 'Black Fella's River' or 'Beware of Crocodiles' sprang up around the place. Quite a sight it was too.

Anytime from 6 am through to midnight, if anyone dropped by, Old Bill was there to welcome them, dressed as he always was in his long Royal Flying

Doctor T-shirt, shorts and a pair of ripple-soled desert boots without laces. And he'd greet everyone by calling them either 'sonny' or 'lass' or 'girlie'. It didn't matter who you were or if you were twenty or a hundred, a pauper or royalty, it was still the same, 'sonny', 'lass' or 'girlie'.

Of course, the moment you arrived you'd be handed a schooner glass of port. It didn't cost anything. Nothing. It was for free. But Old Bill was a crafty bugger. There was a catch. And the catch was that you had to pay to play that board game, the one they have in pubs where the board's had lots of holes drilled into it which have been filled with pieces of rolled paper, and on those pieces of paper there's prizes written. In Bill's case the prizes were souvenirs of the Royal Flying Doctor Service.

When we flew up there to do clinic, Old Bill was invariably booked in for a consultation. Then while the doctor was checking him over, out would come a couple of thousand dollars or so.

'Here, sonny,' he'd say, handing the stash over to the doctor. 'Look after this.'

It was all cash. No receipts. So we can't exactly tell just how much Old Bill raised over the years but it had to be in the hundreds of thousands of dollars, and that was for both the Flying Doctor Service along with the Andamooka Hospital.

They say that Old Bill started his working life as a engineer with the Merchant Navy. When he got out of that, he wanted to go to a place where he didn't have to look at water. Sick of the stuff, he was. Andamooka was the perfect spot and he became very much a creature of his adopted environment. Loved it out there, he did. Why, I remember the day that Old Bill and I were philosophising about life over a few ports.

'Bill,' I said, 'have you ever thought about where you're going to go and what you're going to do when you eventually decide to chuck all this in and retire?'

'Don't yer worry, sonny, I got it all sorted out,' he said. 'First, I'm gonna stay right here, as far away from water as possible.' Then he stopped talking and looked lovingly out over the dry, dusty landscape. There wasn't a blade of grass in sight, not a one. Then he said, 'And as fer somethin' t' do, I reckon I might start up one of them lawn mowin' rounds. I reckon that should keep me more than busy enough.'

That was Old Bill. He had the vision to look beyond the normal plus the wit and cunning to go with it. Like the time he came up with the idea of raffling his caravan as a fundraising venture. He did that for about fourteen years on the trot. Year after year the raffle tickets came out. Mind you, it was the last thing that anyone wanted to win. That caravan was a total wreck. But still, everyone bought tickets. Snapped them up they did. The people didn't mind. They joined in the fun. The reason being, they knew that every cent was going into the Flying Doctor Service.

Another incident that comes to mind was when he was awarded the OAM (Order of Australia Medal). The 'Old Aussie Mug', he called it.

Old Bill McDougall

'Well, sonny,' Old Bill would say, bursting with pride. 'I'm officially an Old Aussie Mug.'

There was a slight hitch with that, though. Old Bill kicked up a bit of a stink when he was told that he had to come down to Adelaide to receive the award. He hated the city. He loathed the city, almost as much as he loathed water. He wanted the Governor to go up to Andamooka to hand over the OAM. At least, then, they could both sit back and indulge in a port or two in a more relaxed environment.

'Cause I tell yer what,' he grumbled, 'I'm not too keen on all that pomp and ceremony they go on with at those sort o' shows.'

Anyway, we finally talked him round and he accepted his fate on the assurance that we'd look after him while he was in Adelaide. That was okay. So, when the time came, we went down to the Adelaide airport to meet him. When the plane landed, off steps Old Bill all decked out in his T-shirt, shorts and desert boots.

'Where's your suitcase?' we asked.

'What suitcase?' he replied. 'I travel light.'

'You can't rock up at Government House dressed like you've just wandered in off the opal fields,' we said.

'Why not?' he reckoned.

Anyway, Jeff Cole who was the General Manager of John Martins at that stage, as well as being on the South Australian Tourist Board, rushed him off to Johnies and decked Old Bill out with a suit and tie, shoes and socks, jocks, the lot. He even had his hair cut and his beard was trimmed. I tell you, he looked an absolute picture of sartorial splendour by the time we dropped him off at Government House.

A few of us had arranged to meet him back at the Grosvener Hotel after the ceremony. Eventually Old Bill arrived looking like a million dollars. We were about to shout him a couple of drinks but when we looked round he'd disappeared. Nobody could find him. Then ten minutes later he appeared with a grin from ear to ear. There he was — he's got his old T-shirt on, his desert boots, his shorts and he's as happy as a pig in shit.

'Okay, sonny, your shout,' he announced.

That suit never again saw the light of day.

I tell you, he was a real character was Old Bill. Then later, of course, he got real crook. There were numerous things wrong by that stage, all the results of his free-and-easy lifestyle. I remember the day that we flew him out of Andamooka to bring him down to hospital in Adelaide. The poor old bloke knew that it was his last flight. He knew he was dying. As we were loading him onto the plane, he leaned over and slipped a heap of money to Margo Duke, his great friend from the Andamooka Post Office.

'This is fer me wake, girlie,' he said.

And some wake it was too, I can tell you.

So that's Old Bill, like I said, a real character. He's been dead now for near on eight years. But he certainly hasn't been forgotten because on every Easter

Saturday people from all over set off on the 10 kilometres' walk from Andamooka out to Old Bill's place at White Dam. On the day, they raise six to eight thousand dollars for the Royal Flying Doctor Service. Then when they arrive at the Ettamogah Pub site everyone gathers around and they have a few drinks and a barbecue, all in memory of Old Bill McDougall.

Once Bitten, Twice Shy

I reckon it must have been about four, or half past four, on a Sunday morning. I was still in bed for some unknown reason. Anyway, the telephone rang. It was Big Joe McCraddok, the police sergeant from Birdsville. Mind you, I've changed names and locations here to protect the guilty.

'Come quick. Come quick,' Joe called.

'Why, Joe?' I replied. 'What's the matter?'

'Roota Kozlowski's been bit b' a snake,' he said. 'Roota Kozlowski's been bit b' a snake.'

Now you'd be able to imagine the sort of character Roota Kozlowski was, just from his nickname, but maybe you haven't heard about Big Joe McCraddok. He's quite famous around these parts. A real true-blue bush character. They did an article on him in one of those monthly magazines, a while back. The locals really gave him a stirring about that, especially the way he was posing outside the pub, in his uniform and all. Anyway, that's the media for you. Because, believe me, Big Joe's nothing like that. He's as male as they come; a real man's man, through and through.

'What symptoms has Roota got?' I asked.

'I don't know,' Joe said. 'He's still about half an hour out of town but he's on his way in so, if you come now, you'll be here just that much quicker.'

That sent me into a spin. I mean, Joe of all people knows that it takes time to organise the plane and everything, and there he was expecting me to be in Birdsville at a moment's notice.

'Look, Joe, you'll have to give Roota first aid yourself,' I said. 'I won't be able to get there within half an hour, you know that.'

'Oh,' came the disappointed reply. 'Must I?'

'You've done it plenty of times before,' I said. 'All you've got to do is to apply pressure immobilisation on him the moment he arrives in town.'

There was dead silence.

'Where's he been bitten?' I asked.

The dead silence continued.

'Joe, are you there?' I said. 'Where's Roota been bitten?'

'Look, doc, I can't speak too loud 'cause I'm ringing from the pub. There's a few of the blokes here and all they know is that Roota's been bit b' a snake, but I haven't told them exactly where.'

'But I've got to know exactly where he's been bitten, Joe,' I said, avoiding the question as to what he was doing in the pub with 'a few of the blokes' at that hour of the morning. 'Joe, can you hear me?'

'On the penis,' came the whisper.

Well, that certainly got me thinking. I mean, Roota's Roota and the many and varied stories of his sexual exploits were known far and wide, but how in the hell a bloke could've got himself bitten in that spot defied imagination.

'On the what?' I asked.

'You heard me. Roota's been bit on the penis,' came the answer, fractionally louder.

Well, that was clear enough. It also explained Big Joe's apprehension about having to give first aid. You could just imagine the comments from the blokes in the pub as they watched Joe apply pressure immobilisation to Roota Kozlowski, especially with it being in that particular region. And so soon after the magazine article and all. Joe'd never live it down.

'Look, Joe,' I said, 'I know what's going through your mind, mate, but you've got to forget all that rubbish. The point is, if you don't give the treatment, Roota could well die. Do I make myself very clear, Joe?'

Silence.

'So, Joe,' I continued, 'as soon as Roota arrives, get him to whip down his pants, then apply pressure immobilisation. And what's more, hold onto it until I get there, right.'

Silence.

'Do you hear me, Joe!'

'Okay,' came the reluctant reply.

As the story goes, Roota pulled into town not too

much later, very groggy from the snake bite. He blundered into the pub and saw Joe over by the bar with a few of the blokes, all of them looking extremely downcast.

'Have yer spoken to the doctor?' Roota asked.

'Yes,' Joe mumbled.

'What did he say?'

'Well, Roota,' Joe said, 'doc reckons yer gonna die.'

One Shot

This happened in a place called Boulia, which is 140 nautical miles south of Mount Isa, in the Diamantina channel country. And as in many of those places out that way, they've got very wide main streets. That's because, in the olden days, they needed a hell of a lot of room to turn the bullock wagons around. Later, of course, they came in handy if there was some emergency or other and you needed to land your aeroplane in the town.

Boulia was such a place.

To paint the scene, it's big sky country, not many trees, dead flat. You can see forever, and, as evening nears, it takes a long time for the sun to go down. It seems to just hang there, inching its way down to the horizon. Then all of a sudden, poof, and it's gone. There's very little twilight under those conditions.

Anyway, it's late afternoon in Boulia and there's this guy and his wife, or de facto, who'd had a few too many drinks in the pub and they have this doozey of an argument, a real donnybrook. 'F'n this and f'n' that.' All the accusations, the incriminations, the whole works. The upshot of all this is that this woman storms out of the pub. 'I'll give yer a lesson yer'll never forget, yer bloody so-and-so,' she says.

'Yeah, yeah,' the bloke slurs in a smart-arse manner. 'Yer wouldn't have the guts.'

But little did he know that she's on her way home to get the .22 rifle. So she grabs the gun and comes back and waits on the diagonal corner about 150 yards down-sun from the pub.

Eventually, the bloke wanders out. And remember how I was saying that it takes a long time for the sun to set? Well, there he is, with the sun at his back, and he can see this woman with the gun as clear as day. Conversely, she can't see him too well because the sun's shining straight into her eyes. But she knows it's him. She knows it's the guy. And it's her full intention to shoot in the general area of the guy, just to put the wind up him, like, to give him the lesson that she said she'd give him.

So he starts to move towards her, holding his hands up, and she lifts the gun to her shoulder and takes aim. No doubt she's still a bit pissed, like. So then she pulls the trigger. Bang. One shot. Straight through the guy's head.

Soon after, we get the call in Mount Isa. Now the doctor reckons that most gunshots turn out to be fatal. 'Look,' he says, as we rush out to the aeroplane, 'if he dies, it then becomes a police matter and it's no longer got anything to do with us.'

But the report comes through from the nurse at Boulia that this guy is still alive. So there we are — I've done all the checks. The engines are warming up. Everything's just right. And I'm just about to open it up and head down the runway when the doctor gets a call through on the HF long-range radio.

'Hang on,' he says.

So I stop.

'He's gone.'

So I kill the take-off.

Pass the Hat

One of the first fundraising appeals for what was then known as the Australian Inland Mission happened back in November 1928. It was on that date that old Jock McNamara passed his hat around the front bar of Mrs Palmer's pub in McKinlay. And, what's more, he made a few quid too, or so I heard.

At the time old Jock owned Squirrel Hills Station which was situated halfway between McKinlay and Boulia, out in the north-west of Queensland. One day he and his son-in-law, Tom Lucas, were out mustering cattle in the Selwyn Ranges. Now, for those who don't know, the Selwyn Ranges consists of some very rugged and mountainous country, most of which is impassable by vehicle. Anyway, old Jock was climbing through a particularly rough patch on his horse when all of a sudden the rubble gave way. The horse reared. Up it went, it lost its balance, toppled over backwards and 'thud' down it came smack-bang on old Jock, squashing him and breaking his pelvis among other things. Very badly injured he was. Couldn't move.

Now this happened before pedal radios existed. Alf Traeger came up with the first of his radios a year later, in 1929, so there was no way that Tom could call for help, not from out in the middle of the Selwyn Ranges, that's for sure. What's more, there were no telephones out that way either.

So Tom dragged old Jock under the shade of a tree. 'Here, Pop,' he said, 'here's some water and a bit of food. I'll go and see if I can get some help.'

And that's where Tom left old Jock, propped up under a tree, out there in the Selwyn Ranges, with some water and food and a gun to keep the dingoes at bay. Then Tom rode for ten hours straight until he came across a mustering camp. Mind you, that was still out in the middle of nowhere, but when he told the head stockman about old Jock's accident the bloke offered to drive him into McKinlay, which was where the nearest telephone was.

When they finally arrived, Tom went straight to the McKinlay Post Office where he rang through to the Australian Inland Mission in at Cloncurry and gave them the details of the accident and the general location of where he'd left old Jock.

'We'll be there as soon as we can,' the AIM Flying Doctor said.

Now the actual plane that was used for the evacuation was imported by Hudson Fysh of the then Queensland and Northern Territory Aerial Service, later to be known as Qantas. That happened back in 1924. It was a De Havilland DH 50, a single-engined four-seater biplane where the pilot sat in an outside cockpit. John Flynn had leased the DH 50 for two shillings per mile, plus a pilot, a chap called Arthur Affleck, and two engineers. There's a big model of this very same aeroplane in Cloncurry, if you're ever up that way.

Anyway, that aside, having now alerted the Flying Doctor, Tom jumped back into the truck and they drove to a nearby station where they organised an old iron bedstead to be used as a stretcher. Then along with a couple of volunteers they headed back out to old Jock. When they'd driven as far as they could into the Selwyn Ranges, they grabbed the bedstead and set off by foot.

By this time Arthur Affleck, the pilot, had landed the small plane on an open patch of country, still many miles from the accident scene. But it was as close as he could get with the DeHavilland. Now the doctor on that trip was a Kenyan chap by the name of Dr K St Vincent Welch. He was the world's first Flying Doctor, meaning that he was the first doctor employed by the Australian Inland Mission. Anyway, Dr Welch grabbed his gear and along with Arthur they started to walk in the direction of where old Jock was supposed to be.

While Dr Welch and Arthur were on their way, Tom and his helpers had reached old Jock. As you might well imagine, after having been stuck out there for almost two days the old fellow's condition had deteriorated somewhat, but he was still alive and that was the main thing. So they laid him out on the bedstead, latched onto an end each and they set off, back out of the Selwyn Ranges.

Tom Lucas and his crew travelled for what was left of that day and into the night until, as luck would have it, they stumbled across Dr Welch and Arthur. 'Dr Welch, I presume,' Tom remarked. Mind you, he didn't really say that. I just added it in because it sounded appropriate. Anyway, when the doctor saw the agony that poor old Jock was in he gave him an injection of morphine right on the spot. Then, as they headed back to the plane, to save all the time they could Dr Welch kept administering injections as they walked along.

Finally, they got old Jock into the DeHavilland. Now the nearest hospital was at Cloncurry but unfortunately at that particular time there was an epidemic of some sort going through there and so they decided to fly him to the Winton Hospital.

Anyway, to cut a long story short, old Jock McNamara must have been a terribly tough sort of chap because he made a remarkable recovery and, three months later, in November 1928, he came back home to Squirrel Hills Station. Of course, by this time the news of his accident and his miraculous survival had spread near and far. It'd been written up in all the papers as well.

But one of the first things that old Jock did on his return was to go into the local pub, Mrs Palmer's pub it was, right there in McKinlay, and after everyone had welcomed him back he took his hat off and passed it around the front bar.

'Dig deep, fellers, it's for Flynn's Inland Mission,' he said. 'Saved me life, they did. Who knows, it could be yours next.'

'Payback'

I was already really, really tired after having just arrived home off night shift from another flight. Then the call came through. 'We've got a Code One Emergency out at Nyrippi,' they said. 'A guy's unconscious with a GCS of three.'

Now a GCS, or Glasgow Coma Score, is the way that head injuries are rated and, among other things, is gauged on your best verbal response, eyes opening, and your best motor response. If there's nothing wrong then your score is usually fifteen. If it's under nine you've got a serious head injury. Having a three wasn't a good sign really; more like a life and death situation, with the odds stacked towards death.

Mark, the doctor, Peter, the pilot, and I flew out on that trip to Nyrippi. A sixteen-year-old guy had been cracked over the back of the head by a person wielding a firestick. Apparently the week before the young kid had caused some sort of trouble. This was his 'payback'.

We got out there in about an hour which was pretty

good considering that we had to drive out to the airport and pack some special equipment into the plane. Peter also had to do all his flight checks and so forth before take-off. Anyway, when we landed at Nyrippi the Community Officer was waiting to pick us up. So I grabbed whatever gear I thought we'd need and threw it into the back of his ute on top of his welding gear and bits and pieces of cars and other scrap. Then we headed into the community.

John was the community nurse on duty that night. I think it was his first week at Nyrippi, if not the first night he'd spent by himself out at the community. And he'd done a fantastic job. When the young guy had first come in he'd put a plastic stiff-neck collar on him to keep his neck in alignment. He'd put a drip in, got the oxygen on him, checked his blood pressure, and then rang the Flying Doctor Service in Alice Springs.

By the time he got back from calling us, the young guy had stopped breathing and that's when John started bagging him. So he must have been bagging the patient for at least an hour. By 'bagging' I mean physically squeezing oxygen into his lungs through a mask, virtually breathing for him.

It was amazing. In a hospital, you bag someone for ten minutes and your hands are aching beyond belief. Ten minutes and, like I said, John had been at it for at least an hour. It's heat of the moment stuff. It's all full-on. And John was the only one bagging. There may have been a health worker somewhere but when it's their own family they tend not to want to be hands-on.

What's more, fifteen or so of the family were in the same room watching every move John made, which must've added to the pressure. There were also a few extra police there by that time. They'd driven over from another community because they knew there could be some serious trouble brewing.

So we got into the clinic and Mark said, 'Okay, what's going on?'

'This is the situation,' John said, then explained the medical details and what'd happened.

Then Mark took over which gave John the chance to stand back for a while and catch up with things. Of course, the first thing that Mark requested was mannitol, which is a drug that releases the fluid off the brain. Silly me, of all things to leave back in the plane, I'd left the mannitol. But, luckily, just a few weeks beforehand I'd shown Peter, our pilot, where everything was packed, just in case. So he was able to go back out and grab the drug from the bottom of the cupboard. While Peter was doing that I was getting ready for Mark to intubate by checking the patient's blood pressure and his pupils, and putting up another bag of fluid.

And so we got the young guy intubated, which is sticking a tube in his throat to clear the windpipe. We continued to bag him, though. He was still unconscious. While we were moving him onto a spinal board for the trip back out to the airstrip we got Peter, the jack-of-all-trades, to do the bagging. When that was done, Mark explained the situation to the family.

'Look,' he said, 'he's had a big head injury and he'll probably have to go to the theatre and have an operation.'

After Mark had finished talking, a faint wailing started to rise up from among the women in the room. And as that gathered momentum everyone outside began joining in. This wailing, I don't know if you've ever experienced it, but it's the most haunting sound you're ever likely to hear. It's filled with such pain and sadness that the hairs on the back of your neck go stiff. And there they all were, watching everything that we were doing and wailing at the same time. Louder and louder, all around us.

So we loaded the young guy into the back of the Toyota four-wheel-drive 'troopie' and I hopped in with him. The grandmother and the auntie also hopped in and the two of them kept up this wailing all the way out to the airstrip. Meantime this guy's blood pressure was really low and I was thinking, 'What sort of situation are we in? No one would ever believe this.' And you think — if only people could see what it's like, to be out here in the middle of nowhere, with these poor women wailing and their young boy fighting for his life. It's so scary. It's weird. It's surreal. People just don't believe that you have those sorts of experiences.

By the time we reached the airstrip, about sixty people had gathered from the community. There they were, all just wanting to touch the young guy because they thought that it was probably the last time they'd see him alive. By then the wailing had built up to be a whirlwind. It was like a wall of sound. And it just went on and on and on, spinning around us.

Eventually, the police stepped in and gave us a hand to get the patient onto the plane. One of the family members, a cousin it was, came along to keep the guy company. By that stage Peter was quite distressed. He'd never seen or heard anything like it. It really got to him.

Anyway, we got the young guy onto the plane and as we were flying back to Alice Springs his heart suddenly faltered. It went into an odd sort of rhythm. And that's when you realise that you're all by yourself. There's no one you can turn to and ask 'What do you reckon about this?' because you're just up there in black vastness. You can't even fax anything to anyone.

It makes you realise just how isolated you are in a situation like that, when you're thousands of feet up in the sky. No one's there to help you. Even when you're being trained in a hospital, they say that if a patient has a cardiac arrest then there'll always be someone to do the airways, someone to do the chest compressions, someone to do the drugs, someone to write it all down and someone else will be there to do this, that and the other. But there we were, just Mark and I, a doctor and a nurse, doing everything we could, and there was this poor young guy, deteriorating further and further.

Still, we managed to get a request through for an anaesthetist to meet us at the airport. Then as soon as we'd landed and got the patient into the ambulance the anaesthetist came and took one look at him. 'Go!' he shouted to the driver. 'This patient needs lots of people focusing on him.'

So the ambos and doctor drove into the hospital with lights and sirens blaring. By that time the young guy was having a cardiac arrest. In the plane I'd noticed that he had a big lump on his temple. It'd sort of swelled up. Like, there was no blood coming from his ears. There was no obvious bleeding from his head. It was all internal.

After the ambos had left, I went back out to clean up the plane. Though he hadn't bled externally, he'd still lost a lot of bloody frothy sputum and there was a mess on the floor. So I cleaned that up. Then I cleaned the equipment. Then I restocked the plane so that it was ready to go again, just in case something else happened.

I must've spent an hour or so cleaning and checking things. By that time it was four in the morning. As I said at the beginning, I was already really tired from a night shift, before the call from Nyrippi came through. But in those sorts of situations your brain doesn't stop and you're always thinking, 'Could I have done something better? Is there something that I didn't see?' Always analysing things.

So on my way home I decided to go into the hospital and that's when I was told that the young guy had passed away.

All the staff were good about it, reassuring me that I'd done everything I could. He'd had an autopsy and it was found that his skull was cracked right across, from one ear right through to the other.

'There's nothing more you could've done,' I was told. 'Even if he was in the neurology unit he still would've died because he'd had such huge internal bleeds.'

But it still upset me. I was also tired beyond belief. But I just wanted to go outside and sit by myself. Just to take my breath. I needed to be alone for a while. So I went outside and I was sitting there, about half-past four in the morning. Everything was quiet, dead quiet. I was tossing things around in my head when a wind blew up from a distance and I swear that it brought with it that haunting sound of people wailing.

Peak Hour Traffic

Bush people are different, you know.

There's two types in our area, out from Broken Hill. First, you've got the sheep people. They're pretty urban sorts because they come to town a fair bit. Then there's the other breed, that's the cattle people. They live right out in the harsh country.

The cattle people don't get to see civilisation too much, maybe once or twice a year, sometimes even less. They're the ones you see around town with the big hats on. Slow movers they are, and they talk in syllables. 'Yeah. G'day. How, yer, goin'? All, right.' That's because, out there, there's not many people for them to mix with, except for their own types. But that's their lifestyle and they reckon it's wonderful, and you can't knock them for that. They probably think that our lifestyle's pretty weird, and you couldn't blame them for that either, especially with all the goings-on you read about in the paper and see on the box.

But it's the isolation that makes the cattle people so unique.

There was an old bloke. His name was Joe. And old Joe was one of the cattle people types. He had been most of his life. He's gone now, God rest his soul. And what you've got to understand here is that there's a lot of these old fellows, just like Joe, who live out on these stations. They don't own the stations, like. They don't even manage the stations. Yet they've lived on the properties for most of their lives, helping out here and there, doing odd jobs, mostly as jackaroos. And a lot of them never get married but they become like family so, when they retire, they just go on living on these stations in a caravan or something.

Anyway, old Joe was a real bushie, retired he was, and he developed a medical problem which we had to keep an eye on. But when we suggested that he move into Broken Hill he dug his heels in.

'There's no way I'm gonna live in a place with street lights,' he complained, and you could tell by the steely look in his eye that he meant every word of it.

So the next best thing we could come up with was for him to move into Tilpa where we flew in regularly to do clinics. Tilpa was the ideal place. There definitely weren't any traffic lights there. Dead quiet it was. It had a population of about eleven, if you can imagine that — just a pub, post office, petrol bowser, that sort of town. But Tilpa had a caravan park, in a manner of speaking. Pretty basic it was. Nothing like the ones you see in the tourist brochures. What's more, it didn't need to be too flash either because you'd be lucky to get one or two tourists coming through every month or so, and that was in peak season.

So old Joe agreed to come in off the station so we could keep an eye on him. Which he did, and he instantly laid claim to being the only permanent resident in the Tilpa caravan park.

As I said, having the problem that he did, whenever we were up there we'd go and visit him in his caravan.

'How yer doing, Joe?' we'd ask.

'Yeah, okay,' he'd say in that real slow bushie drawl of his which didn't give us a ghost of an idea as to how he was really feeling.

Then one day we flew into Tilpa and we noticed that his caravan had gone. It wasn't there anymore. So we asked the nurse, 'Where's old Joe?'

'Oh, he's shifted,' she said.

She told us that he'd moved out of town, down the road a bit. So we shanghaied a four-wheel drive and we drove out of town about 10 kilometres and there's old Joe's caravan, parked well off the road, away out in the scrub. So we knocked on the door of the caravan.

'G'day, Joe. How yer doin'?' we asked.

'Oh, okay,' he drawled.

Then we asked him how his health was, and about his problem, and all that sort of stuff.

'Yeah, okay,' he said, which was a fair bit for Joe, even at the best of times.

Then I asked, 'Joe, how come you've moved out of

the Tilpa caravan park? What're you doing way out here, in the middle of nowhere?'

'Ah, it was the bloody traffic,' he grumbled. 'The bloody traffic in Tilpa was drivin' me bloody balmy.'

Pepper Steak

It's a few years ago now but when I was a Flight Nurse there was one property in particular that we were never too keen on visiting. It was only a smallish place, an outstation, right on the edge of the Simpson Desert.

We didn't drive out there of course, we flew. But on the mornings that we did, we had to be up at the crack of dawn, ready to take off at 6 am, to get to the outstation by 8 am and begin our clinic or whatever. And, as was the routine, when we reached any of these stations we'd circle the homestead a couple of times just to let the people know that we'd arrived and then they'd drive down to the airstrip to pick us up.

Anyhow, on this particular occasion we did just that. We circled the place a couple of times then we landed. The only trouble was — no one came to meet us. No one, that is, apart from the flies. And when I mean flies, I don't mean just the odd couple of hundred. There were swarms of them. Sticky things they were, too.

So there we were, Llew, the doctor, and I, hanging

around in the stinking heat, swamped by these flies, when finally an old EJ Holden station wagon drove up.

'Jump in,' the driver said.

'Where?' Llew asked.

Now this may have sounded like a silly question but for starters there was no back seat in the vehicle. And, what's more, apart from the space where the driver sat, the rest of the station wagon was stacked to the hilt with big pats of cow dung, all at various stages of being dried. Now, when these cow pats were thrown onto a camp fire they might have worked miracles in keeping the mosquitoes at bay, but to the flies they acted like a super magnet. If, as I said, we were swamped by flies when we stood beside the airstrip, we were drowned by the blessed things as we stood beside the vehicle.

With no help in the offing, Llew and I started re-organising these cow pats in an attempt to make some room for ourselves. When that proved to be impossible, we ended up having to perch ourselves on top of this dung the best we could manage. So there was Llew, hanging on for grim life to his doctor's bag full of sterilised gear. There was me, squashed in next to him, dressed in my freshly washed and ironed atomic-blue nurse's uniform. And not only was the inside of the station wagon a sea of flies but I could well imagine a dark cloud of the things trailing the vehicle as we drove through the dust and up to the homestead.

Then, lo and behold, when we got in the homestead

we were tossed a piece of hessian to hang off the verandah for our shade. And so began our clinic, the full medicals, the lot, among the flies and the heat, and in the most basic of hygienic conditions.

While we were checking people over, I could smell kerosene and I remember saying to Llew, 'God, Llew, can you smell that kero?' He just screwed up his nose at the stench and went back to the job at hand.

Not long after that a woman came out and started to set up a fire to cook lunch just a few metres away from where Llew and I were working. I was going to say something to her but I thought better of it. I guess I must have been staring at the massive pieces of pepper steak that were laid out on a plate because she turned around to me and said, 'Would youse people like somethin' ta eat?'

Now the strong smell of kerosene was getting to me so I didn't have much of an appetite. But you have to be very careful not to offend some of these people so I said, 'Yes, just a small piece, please. It looks like very nice pepper steak you've got there.'

'Nothing for me,' said Llew, who was a bit more forthright on the matter.

Anyway, the woman didn't say anything so I continued helping Llew and she got up and disappeared into the homestead. When she came back she was carrying a tin can and in that tin can was some sickly greenish stuff which, to my horror, turned out to be fat. I couldn't stand to look but when she threw the fat into the pan the smell of the bubbling, burning mixture, along with the strong stench of the kerosene, got my stomach in a spin.

'Just a small piece,' I called. 'A very, very small piece.'

But again the woman didn't say anything so I started to walk over to make sure that she'd heard what I'd said. That's when she went to pick up the steak. And that's when it struck me that the pepper bits on the steak weren't pepper bits at all but, in actual fact, all this while the meat had been smothered in flies. Because, as she picked up the meat and threw it into the pan, the flies took to wing. In saying that, I must add that there were a good many who were a bit slow on the uptake and they ended up in the frying pan along with the meat and the bubbling greenish fat.

Llew must have seen my reaction because he came to my rescue like a shot and made the excuse that we couldn't stay for lunch because he just remembered we had an emergency to attend to. So we wrapped up the clinic quick smart and were taken back down to the airstrip in the station wagon which was still stacked to the hilt with cow pats. But we weren't so concerned this time. It was just such a relief to be getting out of there. When Llew and I were dropped off, we said goodbye, loaded the plane and were out of there like a bolt of lightning. Just as well we did, too, because that wasn't the end of the saga.

Later that night the news came through that there'd been a fire out at the homestead. As luck had it, there were no injuries. But, apparently, what I'd been smelling during the day was the kerosene fridge leaking. Then, after we'd left, the fridge blew up and the homestead was burnt down, leaving just the roof and the supports, and no doubt the flies.

'Plonk'

Now this all happened many years ago, so I can't be 100 per cent sure of all the facts. But I was doing an adult education course back in the 1950s and there was this journalist-cum-playwright chap who came to our campus to give us a talk about his travels through central Australia. That would've been some sort of feat back in those days, especially considering that he was driving a small Morris. There weren't any bitumen roads, dirt tracks more like it, nothing but corrugations and dust. It must have been horrendous.

Still and all, as fascinating as it was, especially the way he told it, full of adventure; all about sleeping out under the stars in Central Mount Stuart and the time the Morris got bogged in fine bulldust. Apparently, the only way that he could get the car out was to slide something solid under each of its rear wheels so that he could gain the traction he needed to drive out of the bog. So he hunted around the place and found a strip of corrugated iron which was wide enough to fit under just one of the back wheels. And it was then that he said he realised that he wasn't the only person who'd been stuck in the same spot because painted on that thin strip of corrugated iron were the words 'Now find the other piece'.

Another time he was camping around the site where some blacks had been massacred by whites, back in the 1800s, and to keep his fire stoked up he was absent-mindedly tossing sticks onto it. One stick that he picked up felt different. It was almost smooth, so he had a closer look and discovered that it was half a boomerang. When he later had it checked out he was told that it'd been scraped by shells, so he kept it as a talisman.

But out of all his stories, the one that's stayed in my mind for all these years was told to him by one of the Flying Doctors on his travels. A pretty gruesome story it was, too. It was about a couple of old chaps who'd gone out mining and one of them committed suicide.

Maybe the chap who killed himself had rushed away from some place or other because he'd been let down in love or something, or perhaps he'd done all his dough on their mining venture and they hadn't found a brass razoo. I don't know. That was never fully explained. Anyway, this chap and his mate were apparently tossing down the plonk, the wine like, and the drunker this particular chap got the more depressed he became, until eventually he got a right dose of the miseries.

Anyway, the long and short of it was that he grabbed a knife and ran it across his throat. So his mate got in touch with the Flying Doctor. Frantic he was.

'Oh, God,' he called, 'yer gotta come 'n' see me mate. He's just cut 'is throat. And the blood. You should see the blood. It's terrible. There's blood everywhere.'

And in response the Flying Doctor said, 'Look, keep calm. Get a needle and some cotton and sew it up.'

'But I haven't got a needle and cotton,' called the chap's mate.

'Well,' said the doctor, 'get a bag needle and string.'

'Haven't got that neither,' came the reply. 'Oh, my God, the blood,' the chap kept saying. 'Oh, my God, the blood.'

The poor chap who'd slit his own throat died not long after and, as the story was told to us, the Flying Doctor had to go out to verify the death. So the doctor said to the chap's mate, 'Look, have the grave dug, ready for when I arrive.'

'Okay,' said the chap, 'I'll get a grave ready.'

Anyway, by the time the Flying Doctor got there the other chap had sobered up and had dug the grave. Stone cold sober he was by that time. So the Flying Doctor verified the death. Then, just as they were about to toss the dead chap into the grave, his mate asked in an embarrassed manner, 'Do yer mind if I ask yer something?' he said.

'No,' replied the doctor, 'go ahead.'

'Well,' said the chap, 'I used ta be a butcher, see, and I know all 'bout the interiors of animals. And fer the life of me I've always wondered about the insides o' people, so I was wondering if there was any chance yer could show me some o' the parts.'

'Okay,' said the doctor. He must have been keen to brush up on his surgical skills because he took out a knife and away he went. 'This bit here is the liver.' (Plonk, and into the grave it went.) 'This is the heart.' (Plonk, into the grave it went.) 'And this is the stomach.' (Plonk, into the grave it went.) And so forth and so on until they'd disposed of the body.

And that's the story. Now, as I said, I don't know whether it was exactly true or not, but I can remember that journalist-cum-playwright chap telling us that story to this very day. And each time he said the words 'Plonk, and into the grave it went', you could see all the students' jaws drop that little bit further, mine included.

Rabbit

I heard you on the radio, reading some stories about the Flying Doctor Service, and it reminded me of the time that Mum and Dad were coming over to our place for dinner. It was Dad's birthday and I wanted to cook something special. I'm a pretty good cook, you see, or that's what most people say. But, apart from that, it's something that I really enjoy doing, you know, experimenting with this and that, trying different recipes, different tastes and flavours.

Anyway, I was having a chat to Mum on the phone, discussing plans for the night, and she asked what I was going to cook. I said that I'd planned to start off with some basic nibblies, followed by an antipasto platter, then a seafood soup, and for main course I was going to cook some rabbit.

'Rabbit!' Mum interrupted. 'You're not cooking rabbit, are you?'

'Well, yes,' I replied. 'I've got a really nice recipe for rabbit that an old Italian chap's given me.'

'I don't want any,' she snorted, and then came one of her deathly silences, the ones that she gives when she's digging in her heels about anything.

'Why, Mum?' I asked. 'What's wrong with rabbit?'

Then she told me that when she was a teenager at boarding school, over in Perth, one of her girlfriends invited her to spend the school holidays out on her family's station property. I'm not exactly sure where the station was but, it was away out bush somewhere, south-east of Perth, I think. It was quite a remote place, anyway.

At that stage of her life Mum hadn't been too far from the city and, for the past couple of years, everything that she'd heard from this girl about her parents' station property conjured up images of a romantic life in the outback. There was the freedom of living out in the wide open spaces, the fresh air, the beautiful sunsets, the millions of stars at night, of being able to ride horses from dawn to dusk.

When Mum checked to see if it was okay with Gran and Pop, they were fine about it.

'Go, girl,' Pop said. 'It'll be a great experience.'

So she did.

But, unfortunately for Mum, the experience turned out to be anything but romantic. Quite the opposite really — more like a nightmare. After spending three days cooped up in a sooty old train, when they eventually arrived at the station property Mum found the sparseness of the area to be overwhelming, daunting — frightening even. The air was hot and dusty. Instead of looking in wonder at the millions and millions of stars, she spent the nights swatting millions and millions of mosquitoes. Where her friend stood in awe of beautiful sunsets, Mum was only relieved to know that she'd survived yet another day among the flies. Yes, they did ride horses but, after the first morning, Mum reckoned her behind was so sore that she doubted if she'd ever be able to walk again.

But perhaps what was worst of all was the complete lack of fresh fruit and vegetables. What's more, there wasn't a shop or a green-grocer within cooee.

'Oh,' Mum's girlfriend said, 'we get a delivery of fresh food every couple of months.'

Mum must have looked extremely disappointed at that remark because her friend was quick to add, 'Don't worry, Margaret, the next delivery's due in a couple of days' time.'

The mere thought of sinking her teeth into a nice, crisp apple was the only thing that kept Mum going. So she suffered through the lack of fresh vegetables and fruit. She suffered through the desolation. She suffered through the heat and the dust. She suffered through the flies and the mosquitoes. She even attempted to get back on a horse, but she fell off.

Then, the day before the delivery of fresh food was due, the storm clouds rolled in, the sky opened and down came the rain. Mum reckoned that she'd never seen the likes of it, still to this day. What's more, the rain didn't look like stopping. It kept bucketing down. And with the soil out that way being sand and clay, or whatever, the water just built up and up. The creeks burst their banks and they got flooded in so bad not even a horse could get in or out.

To start with there was still a little food remaining. But, after a week, things were getting pretty desperate. Then the week after that they were in real trouble. That's where the rabbits came in. They'd been flushed out of their warrens and had scrambled onto the only piece of available land they could find, which was around the station homestead.

Poor Mum. If one of her major gripes was the inferior quality of the food, by the third week her staple diet consisted of not much more than dried bread, black tea and rabbit, rabbit, rabbit and more rabbit. Mum reckons that they had boiled rabbit, roasted rabbit, minced rabbit, fried rabbit, rabbit portions, fricassee of rabbit, rabbit stew. They had rabbit every-which-way, day in, day out, and still the water didn't look like receding.

'Without a word of a lie,' Mum said, 'there were so many rabbits that you could sit on the back doorstep and just about shoot the blessed things with your eyes shut.'

So there they were, out in the middle of nowhere, surrounded by a sea of water facing the choice of either starving or eating more rabbit. Mum said that it even reached the stage where starving looked like being the better of the two options.

Then one morning as Mum and her friend were lying around in bed, thinking about making a move, they heard a plane fly overhead, really low it was.

'It's the Flying Doctor,' the girl's father shouted from the kitchen.

They were up in a flash and everyone raced out onto the verandah. And it was, too. It was the Flying Doctor plane. Mum thought that it might have been a DC3 or something like that. It was one of those bigger planes, anyway. When the aeroplane did a second fly-over, they threw out a hessian bag stacked full of food.

Mum reckons that she still remembers the meal they had that day. Though it wasn't the nice, fresh, crisp apple that she'd longed for, there was still milk, tinned meat, tinned vegetables, fresh bread and jam.

Everything except rabbit.

Richmond

I'm living in a shed these days. That's where I am now, away out in the bush near Sarina, outside of Mackay. That's in Queensland if you don't know. But it wasn't always like that. I haven't always lived in a shed. Not on your life. I used to own houses, trucks, the lot, but the Public Trust got stuck into me. Took the lot, they did. That was after a semi-trailer cracked my upper jaw and my lower jaw and many other unidentified bones in my skull, along with my collarbone to boot.

That all happened a few years back and now I can't talk properly either, as you might have guessed. It's not only affected my voice. It's gotten to my memory as well so my memory's not quite the same either. Like, I don't know how old I am these days. That's because I used to work the years out by which truck I had at the time. Just like a calendar those trucks were. I used to be a truckie, see, but a semi-trailer got me so I'm nothing now. Then the Public Trust got to me after that and they took everything I owned, the trucks, my two houses, seven acres of freehold land, family heirlooms, two Rayburn slow combustion stoves, my water tanker, pumps, hoses, two caravans, a mobile workshop, the lot. They got everything. I've got all the paperwork here to prove it, if you want to see it.

What's more, they were hoping that I'd die too, but I haven't died yet and I won't for a long time to come, either. You can tell them that as well. I took them through the Supreme Court in the end, and I got them too. It's the principle of the matter that counts. The case might've cost thousands but I got the $110 dollars they owed me. I've got the receipts right here, somewhere. You can have a look at those as well if you like. But that's the Public Trust for you. That's why I live right out here in the shed near Sarina. They can't get me here. You can tell them that too, in your book, if you like.

Anyway, that's got nothing to do with the Flying Doctor Service, has it? But I was just telling you how things are and who to watch out for. That's why I do most of my business by phone, though I write lots of letters about this and that. My mother was born right beside the Combo Waterhole, out past Winton. Winton's the place that Banjo Paterson made famous with that song 'Waltzing Matilda'. There were no doctors out there then. I was born out near Richmond, about 307 miles into the sunset from Townsville.

Anyhow, it might've been somewhere between the mid 1940s and the early '50s, I can't remember exactly. It could've even been before that, maybe. My memory's not the same since the Public Trust got stuck into me. But back then we owned two stations, Rowena and Rolling Downs.

Anyway, it was when I was living in Richmond. I was only a kid then and in those days the main street didn't have 240 volts installed. Some people had their own charging plant but that wasn't everybody. But, also, Richmond had a real wide street, dirt it was, no one out there knew what bitumen was back then. Anyhow, because there wasn't 240 volts there were no electricity poles or anything, no obstructions in the street, and more than once the planes used to land in the main street. Goldring Street it was. I remember that.

I also remember the time that this feller came looking for a woman. He wasn't with the Flying Doctor Service or anything. The plane was called the 'Silver City'. Gee, I remember that too. And he landed just out of town and I led him up Goldring Street. Then when he got to the main intersection he got out of his plane and wandered off to use the telephone. He left the engines going and all. So, anyway, there I was looking after the plane for the chap and the police arrived. I tell you what, they weren't too happy about it either because the propellers were kicking up a mini dust storm.

'Stay away from those propellers, young feller,' the police warned me. 'We don't want to have to collect the pieces of a curious kid who's got chopped into mince by those blades.'

Then there was another time, the one that the

Flying Doctor was involved in. There was a woman. I can't remember her name now. My memory's not the same since the Public Trust got to me. Anyway, this woman was pregnant and it was the wet season and you couldn't drive anywhere because the roads were all mud. Mud was everywhere.

So there was this woman who was pregnant, like I said, and it was an emergency, so the Flying Doctor landed and they came down Goldring Street. I don't know if the police blocked the road or not. Still, there weren't many people there, anyway, not in Richmond at that time there wasn't. But the plane landed. It was either a DH 86 or a DH 84. It wouldn't have been a Goonie Bird, that's what a DC 3 was called. Not many people know that. But I don't think Goonies were around back then. But I'm not real sure. Not since.

Anyway, the Flying Doctor came in and he landed in Goldring Street to pick up this lady, the one who was in the family way. I'm not even sure if she was married or not. I can't remember seeing her wearing a ring. I wasn't looking at that. The Flying Doctor might've had a nurse with him but I'm not sure about that either.

In those days one end of the street sloped down and the other was on a bit of a hill, an up-slope, like. That was called Bore Hill. Naturally, being called Bore Hill, you could get free showers there too, day and night, anytime you like — right out of the bore. Good water it was, too. Not like some of the stuff you get, real brackish.

At any rate, I can't be certain if it actually happened right there on the street or just as they got the woman into the plane but there was a hell of a commotion and I couldn't see anymore. People were running everywhere, so I asked someone what was going on. 'Hey,' I said, 'what's going on?' And the person told me that the woman had produced a baby.

Then as the plane zoomed up Bore Hill and took off on its way to Cloncurry, apparently she produced another one. So she had twins, like. Anyway, I don't remember what their names were but I reckon that the woman might've called one of them Richmond or something.

Run and Catch

You've got to remember that at that stage my wife, Penny, and I were in our mid to late twenties. We were totally invincible. Nothing could happen to us. We'd go out and do anything. It really didn't matter. It was just one of those things. It was a job that you just had to do because people needed you. So you went and did it. And of course with the RFDS pilot and nursing sister living together, as a team we were simply brilliant. The phone would ring and I'd elbow Penny in the side and say, 'Come on, we've got to go.'

Like the night we went to pick up that guy out of Wyndham. They phoned around midnight. 'We've got a bad one here,' they said. So I gave Penny a nudge and we were out of bed in a shot and into the plane in about twenty minutes. I fired the monster up, then we went like a bat out of hell for Wyndham.

What had happened was that there's this very beautiful little place at Wyndham called The Grotto. It's a waterhole set in steep granite walls and cliffs rising to about 100 feet high. It's completely sheltered, and it's always running with crystal clear water which is gorgeously cool even in the middle of the hottest day. Everybody used to go swimming there.

Anyway, these people got full of booze and wandered out there at night. Then this guy decided that he'd take the easy way down so he dived off the top of the cliff. The only drawback was that he landed in about two inches of water.

Honestly, it was like picking up a bag of jelly. It was terrible. Shocking. We never did much of what they call 'stabilising' in those days. It was all 'run and catch' where we picked the patients up and flew them to a hospital as quick as we could. And this guy had broken everything that it was possible to break.

Then when we got him on board the aeroplane, they said, 'Look, you're going to have to take him to Perth.'

'Bullshit,' I said, 'he'll never make it to Perth. Call Darwin and tell them we're coming.'

'No, you can't go to Darwin,' they argued. 'Darwin won't accept you.'

'Pig's arse, they won't,' I said. 'Just tell 'em we're coming.'

So I took off and headed straight to Darwin and we put down on the airstrip just as dawn was breaking. Thankfully an ambulance was there to meet us. As we unloaded this guy I said to Penny, 'Well, Pen, we'll never see him again.'

Three months later he walked off a Fokker Friendship back in Wyndham. Absolutely, bloody unbelievable.

Skills and Teamwork

Being a doctor, a lot of the stories that I have are of a medical or technical nature. They're not real humorous so I'm not sure that they'll have much appeal. I'd just like to say that if anything exemplifies what the Royal Flying Doctor Service is about, it's skills and teamwork. No one along the line of operations is either more or less important than the other. It doesn't matter if you're a doctor, a nurse, pilot, radio technician, engineer-mechanic or whatever, we've all got our own particular skills. We've all got to pull our weight. If one link in that chain falters, so does the whole operation.

I'll give you an example just to demonstrate what I mean. We had a call one day that there'd been a motor vehicle accident out on the Ivanhoe to Hay road, about 80 plane-kilometres from Ivanhoe. The police who were at the scene informed us that there were two very critically injured people and one who was not so bad.

The problem was that there weren't any airstrips

SKILLS AND TEAMWORK

nearby so we either had to motor the injured out or we had to get in there somehow and land on the road.

Now, there's certain criteria for landing on a road. Firstly, it has to be declared an emergency and has to be approved by the Aviation Safety Authority. Then there must be a straight stretch of road of at least two kilometres. It must be more than amply wide enough. All the guard posts have to be knocked down. No culverts. The camber of the road must be such that it won't affect the safety of the plane's landing. The road must be blocked at either end by the police. Also the wind has to be in the right direction, that's as well as the usual landing conditions.

Normally, we only take one crew in the plane, along with the pilot. A crew consists of a nurse and a doctor. But in this case the injuries were such that we decided to take two crews. That made a total of five people, including the pilot.

Then as we were about to land we were informed that one of the victims had just died. This caused us to have a rethink about the situation, taking into account the high risk involved in landing on a road at the best of times. But there was still one patient down there who was in a critical condition so we decided to go ahead.

When we landed, and very successfully I might add, it struck me just how skilful the pilot was. It was an impressive feat. He'd just taken a King Air plane worth four to five million dollars, weighing five tons or so, with five of us on board, and landed the thing dead square at 180 kilometres per hour on a bush road. What's more, I noticed later that he had only about 18 inches (that's 30 centi-metres) to spare on each side of the plane's wheels to the verge of the road.

That's what I mean about skills. Amazing.

Still and all, in that particular case things didn't turn out well. The remaining critically injured patient unfortunately died while we were attempting to resuscitate him. We were able to fix up the not-so-injured person without too much problem. In that patient's case, time wasn't such a vital factor. So the police took us all into Ivanhoe, leaving the pilot free to take off with an empty plane — because of the safety factor once again.

So, as I said, the Royal Flying Doctor Service is all about working as a team where everyone uses their own particular skills to the best of their abilities.

Everyone relies on each other and, even then, you can have all the skills, expertise and teamwork in the world but time's against you. It's especially sad when there's young children involved.

That's a real tragedy, a tragedy beyond words.

Snakes Alive!

There was one poor fellow who lived out near Lake Stewart, up in the far north-western corner of New South Wales.

Anyway, it was a very hot night. The moon was full. As bright as a street lamp, it was. This fellow and his wife were sleeping outside in the hopes of catching any breeze that might happen to drift by. During the night he rolled over, and that's when he felt something scratch his back, razor sharp it was. Initially, he thought it was the cat but, when he turned over to shoo the thing away, he made out the deadly form of a snake slithering off in the direction of the chooks' coop. So he dashed inside, got his shotgun, charged back outside, and started firing into the chooks' coop in an attempt to kill the snake before it got away.

Of course, all this noise woke his wife. When she saw her husband blasting away into the chooks' coop, with her precious hens flying left, right and centre, and him calling out, 'I'll get yer, yer dirty bastard!', she drew the conclusion that the poor bloke had finally cracked. He hadn't been himself lately. What with the extreme isolation, the extreme heat, the extremely full moon, and the extremities of their current economic concerns — all these things had eventually caused him to go off his rocker.

So there was this chap's wife telling him off, yelling at him to stop slaughtering her chooks and him still blasting away, mumbling something about how he was trying to kill a snake that'd just bitten him.

'Well, where's the snake then?' she shouted.

He stopped firing and when the dust had settled they peered through the moonlight. No sign of a snake. So he showed her his back. The wife took a look and saw a couple of deep scratch marks.

'You've been scratched by the cat,' she said.

'It were a snake,' he replied.

'A cat,' she said.

'A snake,' he replied.

This went on for a while, with his wife arguing that he'd been scratched by the cat which, in turn, had caused him to lose his marbles and shoot up her chooks, and him declaring that he was in full control of his marbles and that a snake had bitten him and, what's more, he'd seen it slither into the chooks' coop which was why he was shooting in that direction.

With both of them finally agreeing to disagree, he put in a call to the Flying Doctor. The doctor advised that the best thing for him to do was to drive into Tibooburra and get the nurse to have a look. 'Okay,' he said and he headed off to Tibooburra, leaving his wife behind to tally up the dead in her chooks' coop.

But his troubles didn't stop there. By the time the chap got to Tibooburra the snake venom had started to take effect. So when the nurse was disturbed at some ungodly hour by a bloke with a very slurry voice banging on her door, she assumed that he was drunk. It'd happened before. Blokes getting a skinful and knocking on her door. Usually, they weren't too much of a problem. All she had to do was tell them to get lost and they'd wander off, most of the time not knowing what they'd done in the sober light of day.

But this drunk was different. No matter how many times she told him to get lost, he still wouldn't budge from her door. Then when the chap started ranting and raving about how he needed to see the nurse because his wife didn't understand him, she rang the police.

So before the chap knew it, he was being apprehended.

'Yer got it all wrong. I've been bit b' a snake,' he protested groggily.

'That's the best one I've heard in a long time,' replied the policeman.

While all this kerfuffle was going on, the doctor had been attempting to get through to let the nurse know that the chap coming in from Lake Stewart had a suspected snake bite, and could she keep him under close observation. The problem was that the nurse didn't hear the call. It was only after the chap had been carted off that the doctor made contact. Yet, even then, the nurse didn't twig. In fact, during the conversation she complained to the doctor about the hell of a night she was having. How it was as hot as Hades and then, just as she had finally got to sleep some drunk started banging on her door and she'd had to call the police to come and cart him off.

Anyway, the chap went from bad to worse during the night which caused everyone to reassess his situation and he was flown to hospital the next day.

Nearly died, he did.

Spot on Time

It turned out to be the most wonderful experience. But it certainly didn't start that way, especially with a neighbour's wife ringing me one night, from out past Rawlinna, saying that her husband had come a cropper off his motor bike.

'Well,' she said, when I asked about the extent of his injuries, 'fer starters, all his head's scalped back, like.'

This didn't sound too promising for the bloke, not at all. What's more, I surmised that the chap had received multiple head injuries, which proved to be right. The thing was that, as a nurse, I could only do so much. For him to get the proper treatment for the injuries he'd sustained we had to get him into a hospital, and as soon as possible.

Timing was always going to be the critical factor as to whether he lived or died. So I got in touch with the Flying Doctor at Kalgoorlie and asked them to fly out to Haig immediately — Haig was the closest airstrip to the chap's homestead, out along the railway track. The problem then was that it'd take me at least two hours to drive out to the property along the railway service road, then bring the patient back to Haig to meet the plane. Mind you, out along the Nullarbor the service roads are terrible travelling at the best of times.

But luck was with me. The Road Master at Rawlinna stepped in and offered his help. And that's what saved the bloke's life. See, the Road Master had a Toyota Hilux which, as well as having normal tyres for road use, had also been specially fitted with steel wheels so that it could run on railway tracks. So he put the Toyota up on the hydraulics gismo, which was situated under the vehicle, and jacked it down on the railway track.

Just before we headed off I asked my hubby to gather everyone together and go out to Haig and light the airstrip with little kerosene lanterns — 'flares' we call them — so the plane could see where to land.

The next thing I knew we were hurtling along the railway track at a 100 kilometres an hour with the Road Master fiddling around, getting things ready to place the injured chap in.

'Look, no hands,' he said as a sort of joke. He must have seen the shock on my face because he was quick to add, 'Don't worry. It's so flat out here that, from when you first see a train's light until it reaches you, well, you can allow a couple of hours at least.'

Anyway, that particular problem didn't arise because within twenty minutes we were as close to the injured bloke's homestead as we could get by rail. So the Road Master lifted the Toyota off the track and onto its normal tyres ready to drive the couple of kilometres to the homestead.

When we got there the bloke was a real mess, worse than what I'd first imagined. Things were touch and go. I patched him up the best I could and we put him in the back of the Hilux before we transported him back across country to the railway line. That was the roughest part of his journey. Once we were there the Road Master put his vehicle back on the railway track and we headed off the 30 or so kilometres to Haig.

I must say that I was deeply concerned for the life of the accident victim. But just as we about to take the Toyota off the track at Haig, a bright light appeared in the sky, out to the north. I forget who was helping me in the back of the vehicle, but I remember saying, 'God, what're those lights?' Then it dawned on me. 'Oh hell,' I said, 'it's the plane. It's just coming in to land!'

So we dropped the wheels again and drove straight out to the airstrip. I tell you, with all the turmoil of that particular night, the arrival of the plane couldn't have been more spot-on. It was like we'd rehearsed it a million times over. Then when the doctor got out of the plane, a female it was, she must have been pretty new to the game, well, she reckoned that the scene looked like something out of the television show 'The Flying Doctors'. There it was, about half-past eleven, twelve, at night, and there were all the neighbours who'd come along to help light up the airstrip with flares.

So they flew the bloke straight out to Perth where they fixed him up. And though he had a really bad time of it, with long-term memory loss and what-not, he's as good as gold now. No problems. He's got two more kids and, what's more, he's back on the job, riding that bloody great big motor bike of his, the same one that bucked him off.

Squeaky the Stockman

It was a hot, still Sunday in Nappa Merry when Squeaky the stockman and his mates began maintenance work on an old Southern Cross windmill.

As usual, Squeaky somehow managed to draw the short straw and was given the job of climbing to the top of the windmill to oil the blades, grease the bearings, and so forth. There he was, working away, when a gust of wind came out of nowhere. The blades of the windmill suddenly spun into motion and Squeaky was knocked clean off the top platform. Down he fell in a flail of arms and legs.

For those who don't know, it's a good distance from the top of a windmill down to ground level. In this case, the only thing in the way was a water delivery pipe, about a yard or so off the ground.

The rest is history.

Some say that the pipe saved the wily stockman's life. But at what pains, I ask. Because a split second before impact Squeaky inexplicably parted his legs. Crunch! There he sat, motionless, astride that pipe, a loose leg dangling either side, his mouth rendered ajar, his eyes almost popped out of their sockets.

His workmates rushed to his side. 'How are yer, Squeaky?' they asked. 'Are yer all right, mate?'

But Squeaky didn't say a word. He tried to, mind you, but it was like there was an obstruction in his throat, somewhere just below his Adam's apple, stuck in his oesophagus.

'Ouch,' said his mates as they gently extricated him off the water delivery pipe. After they placed him on the ground, carefully, they called the Flying Doctor.

'Ouch.'

I don't know if you know or not, but Nappa Merry's over in south-west Queensland so it took a while to fly out there. Then just as they'd settled Squeaky into the Nomad aircraft, another call came across the radio. This time a bloke down at Moomba had put a chunk of wood through his leg while chopping a log for the barbecue.

This left the doctor in an awkward situation. On one hand there was the bloke at Moomba who was in desperate need of help. On the other, there was Squeaky. Now Squeaky was a single bloke, a bit on the shy side with women like, but still and all there was the chance that he might want to settle down and raise a family some day. If so, an emergency operation might have to be carried out. Time was of the utmost importance and Moomba's in the north-east of South Australia, well out of the way.

'Well, Squeaky,' the doctor said, 'it's up to you,

mate. Are you well enough to make the trip to Moomba before we head back to Broken Hill?'

At that point the wily stockman gave a sort of half-throatal gurgle which the doctor took to mean that he was okay to do the trip to Moomba.

'Brave decision,' the doctor said, before loading Squeaky up with pethidine, just in case the pain caught up with him somewhere along the way.

So they arrived in Moomba and picked up the bloke with the chunk of wood through his leg. The doctor gave the Moomba chap a shot of pethidine, plus an extra shot to Squeaky, just in case. As they were about to take off, lo and behold, another call came through. This one was from my wife who'd contacted them to say that I'd scalded my arm and was in need of emergency treatment.

Now the bloke with the lump of wood through his leg was no real problem. He could wait. But Squeaky . . . Squeaky was a different matter.

'Well, Squeaky,' the doctor said, 'it's up to you, mate. Do you reckon you're well enough for another diversion before we head off back to Broken Hill?'

Squeaky gave another half-throatal gurgle, which the doctor took as an assurance that he was okay to do the trip from Moomba over to our property, just south of Broken Hill, before heading to the hospital.

'Brave decision,' the doctor said, then loaded Squeaky up with another dose of pethidine, just in case.

The doctor radioed ahead explaining the situation

and asked if I could be ready to board the aeroplane as soon as it landed. So my wife drove me to the airstrip and the moment the plane cut its engines I jumped aboard. But when the pilot attempted to boot the engine of the Nomad, it was as dead as a doornail. He tried again. Same result. Dead silence. All we could hear was Squeaky letting go with one of his gurgles.

'We'll have to call out another plane,' said the pilot. 'The Nomad's buggered.'

So my wife drove us back to the homestead to escape the heat until the reserve plane arrived. There the doctor pumped some more pethidine into us all, just to tide us over.

Now perhaps it was because of the pethidine, I don't know, but soon after, Squeaky began to lighten up. Not that he could talk, mind you, but his throatal gurgles began to rise in pitch. So much so that by the time the reserve plane landed, Squeaky was sounding like he'd had a triple overdose of helium.

'Squeaky, yer getting squeakier and squeakier,' the pilot remarked.

Now I know it wasn't much of a joke. I guess you had to be there at the time, but it was enough to get Squeaky, me and the bloke with the lump of wood through his leg giggling like little kids, which was something we continued to do right up to the time we arrived at Broken Hill Hospital.

I don't know what happened to Squeaky the stockman after that. We sort of lost contact. He went one way and I went the other. So whether or not his family jewels needed rectifying, I don't know. But that was a fair while ago now and he still comes to mind occasionally — oddly enough, when I think about him I can't help but wince a little.

Stowaway

There was an accident in the middle of the night. A car had turned over with two people in it, a husband and wife. The husband was dead. The wife, who was the passenger in the vehicle, was still alive but in an extremely critical condition.

It was touch and go.

We flew to the nearest town immediately. As I said, it was in the middle of the night so they had to line the runway with flares. It was a bit hairy there for a while but we landed and the ambulance drove out to meet us. We loaded the woman into the plane. Then the problem arose as to what we'd do with the husband's body.

We looked blankly at each other for a while until the ambulance fellow asked if we'd be able to take it back in the plane with us. Of course we could see the logic of the request. Taking the body back home with us was the most practical and economically feasible thing to do. The funeral was to be held there so it'd save another trip out. But, naturally enough, our doctor wasn't keen on having the body in the aeroplane in full view of the wife.

'She's critically ill and extremely distressed,' he reasoned. 'If she saw her dead husband it could be a turning point and she could give up hope and go the same way.'

The only thing that we could come up with, to get around the problem, was to stow the body in the rear luggage locker of the Nomad aircraft. The problem was, the luggage locker wasn't large enough to take the body lying down. So we got the ambulance fellow to give us a hand to get the husband's body into such a position that it'd fit inside the locker. In this case, we were forced to squash him up into a crouched kneeling position. After we got the husband safely stowed away in the luggage locker, we then took off to the nearest city where the wife could receive emergency treatment.

I'd say it took us about an hour and a half to get to the city. Turbulence was minimal, which was lucky. It's distressing enough to go through a rough patch inside the plane itself where the air pressure is equalised and you've got safety belts on to minimise the bumpy ride. But there's no such luxury in the luggage locker, and the last thing we wanted was to have the body thumping around in the back.

Things went quite smoothly. When we'd landed, the ambulance was waiting and the woman was rushed to hospital where she eventually went on to make a full recovery. But we were left with a problem out at the airport. With the wife now not in the plane, it would have been far better to have had the husband's body in with us for the return trip. We all agreed on that. But it was a busy airport and, if anyone saw us dragging a body out of the rear luggage locker of a Nomad aircraft, a few questions might be asked, questions that we weren't too keen on answering, considering the delicate situation.

Eventually, we decided to leave the body where it was, just in case. So we departed the airport to fly back to our base. That trip took us about another hour and twenty minutes, and once again we were relieved by the lack of turbulence.

Anyway, we arrived back home quite exhausted from all our travels, only to be confronted by the undertaker. Now the undertaker was a very pedantic man, as most undertakers seem to be. Everything had to be just right. There he was, the coffin at the ready, all organised for the body to be placed in, nice and snug and neat. Apparently, he'd been waiting for a fair while so he wasn't in the best of moods to start with but worse was to follow. See, the rear luggage locker of the Nomad isn't heated so the temperature during the flight got down below minus 2°. Not only that but a few hours had gone by since the chap had died.

'Show me to the body,' the undertaker said in his dry, formal manner.

So we did. We flung open the rear luggage locker and there was the body in its crouched position, frozen stiff and locked solid with rigor mortis.

The Pedal Radio Man

Alf Traeger's known as many things — 'the Pedal Radio Man' just for starters. He's also been described as the person who gave a voice to the bush and in doing so connected the more remote areas to the Royal Flying Doctor Service. There's no doubting that Alf was a bloody magnificent technician, I'll vouch for that. The only trouble was that he was the type of chap who wouldn't let anything be. He was always fiddling with the radios, trying to improve them, and that's what drove us up the wall.

After the five watt pedal radio was established in the bush, Alf started working on a couple of modifications. The thing with all those radios — and there were a couple of hundred or so in the network back in 1950–51 — was that someone had to service them, right. Frank Basden, the radio operator at the Broken Hill base, did some, as did Alf himself, which caused us all the headaches.

But those chaps like Alf and Frank weren't travelling around anywhere near as much as we were. So each time Vic Cover, the RFDS pilot, and I used to do the rounds of the stations we also did a bit of servicing on these radios, when the need arose. Vic knew a lot more about them than I did. But the thing that we came up against very smartly was that if Alf had had his hands on them after they'd been installed, the circuit diagram on the inside of the sets never matched the wiring because he'd gone and changed things about.

Anyway, the ones that we couldn't fix on the spot, we used to cart back to Frank Basden who, as I said, was the radio operator at the Broken Hill base, and Frank would have a go at fixing them. By this stage Frank had been with the Flying Doctor Service for about twenty-five or thirty years and he knew Alf Traeger very well. Frank was an interesting fellow too. He's dead now, unfortunately. A very knowledgeable chap, he was. He had to have been to be able to follow Alf's so-called 'modifications'. Anyway, apart from fixing these radios on the base, Frank also gave advice over the air if someone out on a station was having problems.

When Vic and I told Frank about the fun and games that we were having with the radios Alf Traeger had fiddled around with, he just laughed.

'You reckon that Alf drives you blokes bloody balmy,' he said. 'I'll tell you a little story. Do you know the bloke who was at Pincally Station, the one with the droll sort of voice?'

'Yes,' Vic and I said.

'Well, he got on the radio about the same sort of problem that you're having with the circuit diagram. "Ah," he said, in that voice of his, "are you that bloody Frank Basden bloke?"'

'"Yes, I'm Frank Basden,"' I said.

'"Well, Frank,"' he said, "I've got a bit o' bloody trouble here with the 44-metre frequency, 'n the 78's not all that bloody good neither."'

At that time there were three available frequencies, the 44, the 78 and the 148. The 148 didn't carry very well with those little radio sets and we had to rely upon people relaying the messages which, of course, they did, and everybody within range used to tune in and listen in to the message. That's why the 148 was ideal for the 'galah sessions' where all the ladies used to get on and talk to each other. Worked perfectly for that. What's more, the whole network used to come alive as soon as the doctor got on the air.

'Then the chap from Pincally says, "Frank, I had a go with the bloody screwdriver last night and I think me radio's buggered."

'"What did you do?" I asked.

'"Well, I took the bloody guts out'a the middle'a the thing to see if there were anything wrong and everything looked like it were hooked up proper."

'"What do you mean, Pincally," I said, "by saying that you took the guts out of the radio?"

'"Well, I undid that big round piece, you know, the bloody one that's got all them little contacts on the outsides because it wasn't turnin' around, 'n I thought that it might'a been the trouble but it wasn't 'n now the whole thing's in bloody pieces 'n I don't know what to bloody do."

'"Oh, God," I said. "You shouldn't have done that, Pincally, definitely not without the proper authority and advice."

'"Well, I got that, okay," said the chap. "I rang up that Alf Traeger bloke the other day and he said, 'Well, have a go at fixing it yerself, 'n if you can't you'd better get in touch with that bloody Frank Basden bloke. He'll know what to do.'"'

The Telegram

After I left school back in 1950 I spent a hell of a lot of time in the pastoral area out in the west of New South Wales. And around that time the Royal Flying Doctor Service incorporated an online radio service through its base in Broken Hill.

This particular service was greatly appreciated by the station people because they didn't get into town much and it gave them the chance to place orders for food or machinery parts and whatever. In actual fact, I reckon that about 90 per cent of station business was carried out that way, back in those days.

Now, aligned to this online radio service, the Flying Doctor base also ran what us station hands called 'galah sessions'. And these galah sessions were in part set up so that, after the business was concluded, the station women could have a good chat to each other and catch up on all the gossip and stuff. But also, there was some time set aside for urgent telegrams to be read over the air.

Anyway, most of us out on these stations used to

listen in on the galah sessions whenever we could and then to the telegrams as they came through. Everyone used to do it. It was a bit of a lark. What's more, it sort of brightened up our day, hearing the gossip from different parts — who'd had a baby, who was crook, who'd died, who was getting married, and so forth. And also, you never knew when an urgent message might come through for yourself from family or whoever.

Anyway, at this particular time I was working out on the White Cliffs road at Koonawarra Station, just doing ordinary stock work and the like. And we were sitting around one morning listening to these telegrams being read out when we heard what I reckoned to be the daddy of the lot.

Apparently things weren't going too well for one particular family down in Tasmania and there was this telegram which was read over the air to a station hand out at Naryilco Station, in south-west Queensland. I forget the poor chap's name but, anyway, the message said it all and, what's more, with the minimum of words.

It read: DEAR (whatever his name was)
FATHER DEAD — TOM IN JAIL —
SEND TEN QUID.
LOVE
MOTHER

The Tooth Fairy

This is one of Fred McKay's stories. It isn't mine so you'll have to check the details with him.

It happened back in the late 1930s, long before John Flynn died and Fred took over. Fred and Meg had recently been married and they were visiting a cattle station out in the Barkly Tablelands, just over the Queensland border, into the Northern Territory. Anyway, the station's storekeeper-cum-bookkeeper had an abscessed molar, very painful it was.

'Meg'll sort it out,' Fred offered, brimming with confidence in his new wife.

Now, even though she'd completed a two-week crash course in 'tooth extraction' at the Brisbane Dental Hospital before they'd set out, Meg didn't quite share Fred's enthusiasm in her ability. She was new to this rugged bush lifestyle. As you might imagine, it was a big change for someone who was virtually a city girl and she was still trying to find her feet among the dust, the flies, the heat, the cold, the camping out, the cattle, the bore water, the stockmen. Still, she tentatively agreed to give it a go.

But whatever minimal confidence she had completely vanished when Meg arrived at the store. The storekeeper looked a formidable customer indeed. He was a huge man, a mountain in comparison to the 'dental-dummy' that Meg had trained on back in Brisbane. To make matters worse, when the news had spread that a woman was going to have a go at extracting the storekeeper's molar, a crowd of sceptical stockman had gathered, all eager to watch the event unfold.

Until that point in time, Meg had hardly ever pulled a tooth, let alone done it in front of a crowd as rough and as doubting as this mob was. Still, she couldn't turn back now. She'd volunteered her services and she'd have to see it through to the end, whatever that end may be. So she sat the chap down on an old box outside the station store. She gave him an injection and then set to with the pliers or whatever.

Now you might be able to imagine some of the remarks coming from the stockmen when it became obvious that the harder Meg pulled on the molar, the more it seemed that it wasn't going to budge. And the more the molar wouldn't budge, the more anxious the storekeeper became about allowing a woman to attempt to extract his tooth. But if there was one golden rule that Meg had learned in at the Brisbane Dental Hospital, it was 'Once you've got a good grip, never let go.'

So she didn't.

She latched onto that molar and she pulled with every ounce of strength she could muster. Even when the storekeeper started to gargle a protest, Meg straddled him and still hung on and pulled. And when he struggled to free himself from off the old box, Meg clambered up on the box and still hung on and pulled. Then, as the storekeeper attempted to walk away, Meg gave an almighty twist and yank and . . . out came the tooth.

Well, this brought the house down, so to speak. As Meg stood there in complete triumph displaying the molar, the gathering of stockmen exploded into cheers, whistles and applause. But the person that was most stunned was the beefy storekeeper himself. He gazed down upon Meg in complete wonderment and, with the tears pouring down his cheeks and the blood running down his chin, he called out, 'What a woman!'

There's a Hole in the . . . Drum

My father was a pretty tough sort; a roo shooter, on and off, for most of his life, he was.

But back in the days that this incident happened we were living in very isolated conditions, about 60 miles out of Mingah Springs Station, which is about 150 miles north of Meekatharra, in central Western Australia. It was in either the October or November, I'm not sure which, but it was stinking hot and in the middle of a drought, which wasn't unusual way out there.

Anyway, Dad had spent a trying day out building stockyards and it was late in the afternoon when he finally came in. Then just before tea he remembered that he still had to organise some meat for the dogs, so he grabbed his .22 rifle and headed off to kill a kangaroo.

He must have been awfully tired because after he'd shot a roo and sorted it out for the animals, he came

There's a Hole in the ... Drum

back in, put the gun away, had his tea and went straight to bed. Then, early the next morning when he grabbed the gun again, it went off and the bullet went into his stomach, right through his kidneys, and came out his back.

When my mother saw the mess that my father was in, she went into a real tizz. To make things worse, Mum couldn't drive and she was afraid that Dad was going to die before she could organise some help. Anyhow, we did have an old two-way radio. It was one of those ones that ran with the aid of a 12-volt battery. The only trouble was, when Mum went to call for help she discovered that the battery on the radio had gone flat.

Now, to recharge the battery you had to go through a bit of a rigmarole. See, my father had set up an alternator to an old push-bike. And the idea was, when you hooked the flat battery to the alternator and peddled flat out, it'd recharge the thing.

So Mum hooked the battery up to the alternator, jumped on the bike and went like a bat out of hell. Mind you, this was all happening while my father was still sprawled out inside. Then, when the battery was finally recharged, mother took it back inside, wired it up to the radio and started calling the Flying Doctor for help. As I said, she was in a real tizz and with the shock of having to cope with my father being shot, then having to recharge the battery in the growing morning heat, it was all too much. In the middle of explaining the situation to the doctor, she fainted.

Down she went, leaving Dad to struggle over to the radio and complete the call.

As I said, Mum couldn't drive and we lived in a very isolated area. But as luck would have it there was a gentleman, Val Sorenson, who owned Mingah Springs Station as well as Briah Station and he just happened to be visiting Mingah at the time and overheard the call on his radio. Then Mr Sorenson came on the line and offered to come up to our place and pick up my father, then take him back to Mingah which had the closest airstrip to where we lived.

'Yes, please,' my father said.

So Mr Sorenson jumped into his old open-top jeep and drove the 60 miles up to our place. That trip took a fair amount of time because there wasn't really a proper road between Mingah and our place. In actual fact, it was more like a bush track, and a pretty rough one at that. It wasn't even graded or anything.

When Mr Sorenson arrived a couple of hours later, he loaded Dad and Mum and my little sister into the jeep and they headed back towards Mingah. As I said, it was a hot October or November day and the journey was over a rugged track so Mr Sorenson had to take it extremely slowly. Yet throughout that whole journey Dad remained conscious and kept reassuring everyone that he'd be okay. Like I said, he was a pretty tough sort, especially keeping in mind that almost ten hours was to pass from the time my father had been shot until the time that Mr Sorensen finally arrived back at Mingah Springs Station.

There's a Hole in the ... Drum

Anyway, while they were making their way back down the track the pilot from the Flying Doctor Service arrived at Mingah in his Cessna; or it might have been an Auster, I'm not sure which. All I know is that it was a small plane and there wasn't a doctor on board. But with all the confusion over the radio, with the flat battery and my mother fainting, then my father having to take over in his delirious state, and Mr Sorenson coming in and offering his help, the message hadn't come across very clear at all. So when the Flying Doctor pilot arrived, he fully expected to find my father there ready to be flown straight off to hospital where a doctor was waiting. But of course he wasn't anywhere to be seen.

The pilot then tried to radio through to clear up the situation but he couldn't raise an answer. So he waited for a couple more hours and when it looked like no one was going to turn up he decided that the best thing to do was to fly back to Meekatharra and take things from there. The only problem was that he didn't have enough fuel to get back to the base so he hunted around the place until he found an empty four-gallon drum. He then took the drum and walked the distance over to where the fuel tank was.

But after the pilot filled the drum he discovered there was a hole in the thing and he had to struggle back to the plane with the filled drum while attempting to cover the leak with his finger. It was those extra crucial minutes of delay that saved my father's life because, when the pilot finally reached the airstrip, he drained the fuel into the plane, jumped in and was about to take off . . . and that's when Mr Sorenson's jeep came into sight.

There's a Redback on the . . .

Back in the early 1970s I went to the Northern Territory as a very young and naive school teacher and took up a position on Brunette Downs Station which was then owned by King Ranch, Australia. I was teaching Aboriginal kids there, which was a steep learning curve because, coming from where I did, I soon realised that I had a lot to learn about the Aboriginal culture. But I really enjoyed it, and I still think that we could all learn a lot from the Aboriginal people, particularly as far as caring for family goes.

Anyway, I was in the schoolroom one day and I felt this thing on my neck. 'It must be a fly,' I thought, so I tried to wave it away, like you do. But still the thing didn't move so I gave it a slap. Then when I squashed it, it felt like someone had placed some burning tongs on my neck. When I took a look at the thing, I realised that I'd been bitten by a redback spider.

It was almost lunchtime so I said to the kids, 'Oh look, you can go out for lunch a bit early today.' When they'd gone I went up to the clinic to see the nursing sister. A funny person she was.

'I've just been bitten on the neck by a redback spider,' I said, and she gave me a vacant sort of look.

'Are they poisonous?' she asked.

'Yes,' I said, astounded that she didn't know anything about spider bites.

'Oh,' she replied, 'then I'd better get in touch with the Flying Doctor Service to see what we can do about it.'

'Thanks for all your help,' I said, with a hint of sarcasm.

So I went into my room where I had a first aid book from teachers' college, ancient as it was, and I had a look in that. It said that if you're bitten by a spider the first thing to do is to put a tourniquet on. That seemed a bit ridiculous, especially with me having been bitten on the neck. But by that time I was feeling sick and I was starting to get a fever as well, so I went to bed which, as it turned out, was the best thing to do.

In the meantime, the nurse had been on the radio and explained my situation to the doctor. She was told to treat it like shock and keep a watch for any symptoms. Now what you've got to realise here is that, when anyone's talking over the radio, anyone else can listen in. And they do, quite a lot. So unbeknown to me, my being bitten on the neck by the wretched spider was broadcast throughout the Northern Territory.

Then a couple of months later I went up to this race meeting at Borroloola, which is on the Gulf of

Carpentaria, on the McArthur River. That was a hoot. It's also quite an extraordinary place, mind you. My education continued non-stop while I was up there. Anyway, there was this guy from Mallapunyah Station. A sort of a legend around the area, he was. Well, he came up to me.

'Oh, gee,' he said, in his real droll bush voice, 'so you're the teacher from Brunette Downs, are yer? The one that got bit on the neck b' the redback spider?'

'Yes,' I said, 'that was me. Why?'

And he just stood there, ogling at me, eyeing me up and down from tip to toe. Then finally he shook his head from side to side.

'Jeez,' he said, 'I would 'a liked to 'a been that redback spider.'

Touch Wood

I was a band master at the time and had been sent down to Esperance to get the local brass band started. Anyway there was this vacant brick residence out on a farm, a lovely place it was, and the owners wanted someone living in it, to keep it tidy and so forth. I needed some accommodation so I moved in.

Then I had a heart attack. So they drove me into Esperance Hospital where they got in touch with the Queen Elizabeth Medical Centre in Perth. And the people in Perth said, 'Look, we haven't got any beds just at the moment. You'd better try and keep him alive down there until we can sort something out.'

So I stayed in Esperance Hospital for half a day with the doctors pumping things into me and so forth. Then the message finally came through that there was a bed available in Perth, which was a great relief, I can tell you. But of course, the problem then arose as to how to get me to the Queen Elizabeth Medical Centre post haste. Anyway, to cut a long story short, the hospital got in touch with the Flying

Doctor Service out at Kalgoorlie who were at that very moment getting ready to fly to Perth with a couple of chaps who'd almost killed each other in a pub brawl.

Now the idea of travelling in the confines of a small aeroplane along with two blokes who'd tried to murder each other didn't fill me with too much excitement, I can tell you. So I expressed my concerns.

'Don't worry,' I was told, 'these blokes are so well sedated that they wouldn't harm a fly.'

'Okay then,' I said. 'Count me in.'

So the plane came down to Esperance to pick me up and when it arrived there were these two blokes laid out on the floor, on stretchers. And they were sedated all right, sedated to the eyeballs with alcohol. The plane stank like a brewery. It almost made me crook. Just how on earth they could have inflicted the injuries on each other that they did was beyond the realms of comprehension. But there they lay, completely out to it, both of them severely cut about with glass, 'sedated' to the eyeballs.

Anyway, with the plane being diverted to Esperance at such short notice, the nurse had only enough time to make some quick preparations to accommodate me after they'd taken off. As I said, these two blokes were as full as boots and there was no way that she could get them to budge off the floor. So the next best thing she could do was to set up a little box at the back of the plane, way down the tail end where the fuselage came down in a slope. And that's where I sat, hunched over with my chest almost on my lap, my stomach turning cartwheels from the smell of alcohol, while being hooked up to all sorts of drips and things.

If you think that particular situation sounded uncomfortable, worse was to follow.

'Look,' said the nurse when we were halfway to Perth. 'Look at all that lovely lightning out there. Isn't it exciting!'

'It might look exciting to you,' I replied, swallowing deep.

The next thing, there we were in the middle of a violent thunder-storm and, of course, being down at the rear of the plane was the worst position to be. We were being thrown all about the place. The nurse was stumbling around, struggling to keep all my drips and stuff in. By this stage, not only was my stomach turning over ten to the dozen but a pain started to rise in my chest — not a violent pain, mind you. Still it was just enough to start me thinking, 'You could be in big trouble here, mate.' And throughout this calamitous event, there were these two blokes stretched out on the floor, completely oblivious to the thunderstorm, if not to life itself.

'The only way to travel,' the nurse said at one point, with a nod in the direction of the drunks and, by the way I was feeling, she might have been right, too.

Thanks to both the pilot and the nurse we worked our way through the storms and arrived safely in Perth. When we landed there was an ambulance waiting which whipped me into the Queen Elizabeth

Medical Centre, where I was placed straight on some machinery.

They did the open-heart surgery a day or two later. That was a while back now and I'm still here today and, touch wood, I still will be tomorrow and for a good while to come yet.

Train Hit by Man

Now Barton's an interesting place. Ever heard of it? Not many have. It's a small railway siding out in the Nullarbor, at the start of the world's longest straight stretch of track, leading from there to eternity, then further on to Kalgoorlie. There's bugger-all there these days apart from millions of flies and a fluctuating population of between one and six, and that's counting the stray horses and camels. Even for the most imaginative of real estate agents, the best that could be said about Barton is that it's 'nestled comfortably among endlessly rolling red sandhills'. Beyond that you'd be scratching for compliments.

Back a few years ago when the railways scaled down, there was an old German bloke by the name of Ziggie, a railway worker of some sort, a fettler maybe. Anyway, with all the kerfuffle Ziggie decided to retire after thirty years on the job. But instead of retiring to the Big Smoke of Port Augusta like the rest of the workers out that way did, he thought, 'Vell, bugger it. I've no family, novere to go. Zo as-t long as-t zee Tea and Sugar Train still delivers vater and supplies, I'll stay in zee Barton.'

The trouble was that he'd been left with no place to live. So for the next couple of years he wandered up and down the track with a wheelbarrow picking up the sleepers which had been cast aside during track maintenance. And out of those he built a huge three-roomed bunker, complete with a patio where he could sit and sip on his Milo and watch the sun set over the endlessly rolling red sandhills.

Now you may think that the mention of him sipping on Milo, instead of a gin and tonic or a cold beer or something of a more refreshing nature, was a slip of the tongue. But it wasn't. Old Ziggie drank nothing but Milo. In actual fact, his staple diet was Milo, oranges, potatoes and, as the strong rumour had it, canned dog food. Yep, you heard it right ... canned dog food. Canned dog food, Milo, oranges and potatoes for breakfast, dinner and tea, and a good brand too, mind you.

So Ziggie settled down to life at Barton along with his seven dogs. And he's had a good many more than seven dogs in his time because he keeps a collection of their skulls. If you go to Ziggie's place, the one made out of discarded railway sleepers, there they are, all these dog skulls lined up, along with the empty cans of dog food and the empty Milo tins which he uses as an antenna for his short-wave radio.

But other than being the collector of dog skulls and a connoisseur of fine dog food, oranges, potatoes and

Milo, old Ziggie just happens to be one of the best informed individuals that you're ever likely to meet. As you might imagine, there's not too much for him to do out at Barton except to listen to his short-wave radio, which he does day in, day out. Ziggie knows more about the goings-on of the world than anyone I know. What's more, he has an opinion on any subject and if he doesn't he'll soon make one up.

So life's a pretty solitary affair out at Barton which, in turn, causes the Bartonites to get mighty suspicious when a blow-in lobs into town. Not that many do, mind you. Maybe one or two each decade or so. But just enough for the locals, including Ziggie, to have formed the solid impression that the rest of the world is inhabited by . . . weirdos.

And so it was that one of the locals wandered out at the crack of dawn one day and discovered that some bloke, a blow-in type, had appeared from God-knows-where in the middle of the night and had been bowled over by the Tea and Sugar Train as it was pulling into the siding. The evidence was right there for all to see. There was this complete stranger, sprawled under the front of the train, out to the world, comatose in fact, with his head split open, stinking of grog and looking on death's door.

'Typical of these blow-ins, aye,' someone muttered, to which there was total agreement.

Of course, the train driver was upset. But as he said, 'How the hell could I have bowled someone over when the train only travels at snail's pace?' And there were those that saw his point of view. See, it's been rumoured that the driver of the Tea and Sugar Train wasn't given a timetable upon departure from Port Augusta. Instead, he was handed a calendar because it really didn't matter when he arrived in Kalgoorlie, just as long as he did, at some stage of the year.

Naturally, not long after Ziggie had appeared on the scene he'd come up with a theory about the accident. He reckoned that the train hadn't hit the blow-in, but that the reverse had occurred. In fact, upon closer inspection, Ziggie deduced that the bloke had been so pissed when he'd staggered out of the sandhills and into Barton at some ungodly hour of the night that he'd walked headlong into the stationary train. Crack! Split his head open and down he'd gone like a sack of spuds, right under the front wheels, and hadn't moved a muscle since.

After much discussion the Flying Doctor from over in Port Augusta was called. And while the blow-in lay prostrate under the train, the discussion raged as to whatever reason the bloke might have had to be wandering around the desert in the middle of the night. And so the discussion continued right up until the locals saw the plane land. Then they put a hold on things while a ute was sent out to pick up the doctor and the nurse.

It was during the brief respite that Ziggie organised the making of a bush stretcher. The reasoning behind that was to save precious time so the blow-in could be placed into the back of the ute as soon as the doctor had checked him over. So they slung a bit of canvas around a couple of bits of gidgee then rolled the unconscious bloke onto the stretcher.

When the doctor arrived he went through the full medical procedure. 'This bloke's in an extremely critical condition,' he concluded. 'So, fellers, when you pick up the stretcher take it nice and easy.'

Now, constructing a house out of railway sleepers may have been one of old Ziggie's fortes but making a stretcher out of a strip of canvas and a couple of bits of gidgee apparently wasn't. Because, when they lifted the stretcher, the canvas gave way and the blow-in went straight through and hit his head on the railway track with an almighty thud.

'Holy Jesus,' someone said, 'we've killed him fer sure.'

But almost before those words had been spoken, the blow-in miraculously snapped back into consciousness. What's more, to everyone's surprise, particularly the doctor's, the bloke sat bolt upright. He took one look at the menagerie of faces gawking down at him, then a quick glance out at the endlessly rolling red sandhills.

'Where the bloody hell am I?' he squawked.

'Barton,' came the reply, to which the blow-in got up, shook his head and staggered off down the track, leaving the doctor mystified and locals only more reassured at the weirdness of humankind in the outside world. This, of course, included Ziggie, who wandered back home to tuck into a nice hearty breakfast.

We Built an Airport

It all started when the old airstrip out at Pete May's place was forced to close over winter. For those who don't know, and I guess that there'd be many, Pete May's place is near Elliston which is on the Eyre Peninsula, in the Great Australian Bight. So, anyway, with the airstrip being out of action, it meant that the Flying Doctor couldn't fly in if there were any medical emergencies or if there'd been a serious accident.

We reckoned that it just wasn't good enough. So some people went to Council and complained. They reckoned, and quite rightly too, that either the old airstrip should be upgraded or an all-weather strip be built on a new location. Council agreed in principle but they said that everything was in limbo just at the moment because they were awaiting the outcome of current grant applications to the state and Commonwealth governments. So, when the various governments reckoned they didn't have any money for airstrips and the like, the ratepayers made such a big song and dance about it that a public meeting was called.

An engineer chap came to the meeting with the recommendation that the new airstrip should be placed over the Elliston Swamp which was within half a kilometre from the front door of the hospital. But, without funding, Council said they couldn't afford to go ahead. It was then that the people offered to volunteer their services, vehicles and equipment, on the proviso that Council was prepared to foot the bill for the fuel and maintenance on the vehicles and equipment plus lend us some Council labour.

With Council agreeing to that proposal, the first step was to remove the hills. Blasting started around the end of October. That was a mammoth task in itself, one which caused Council to snaffle every stick of explosive held by all the other councils throughout the Eyre Peninsula.

When the majority of the blasting had been completed we got an expert to come down from Coober Pedy to remove what was left. But because we didn't have the money to pay the bloke, the owners of the motel offered him free accommodation while the pub provided his meals. Another chap came in after that with a stone picker and broke up the rubble.

Then nothing much happened over Christmas, with the harvest in full swing. But straight after harvest the Airport Committee approached various people and community groups in the area seeking their help and support.

Now Elliston's only got a population of just under 300, with around 800 in the district, but within two weeks vehicles and machinery appeared on site. There were about six double-axle tipper-trucks and several smaller single-axles. There were bulldozers, graders, tractors, the whole works. Some started digging out the quarry while others were working on the sandhill. The sandhill itself ran virtually halfway along the proposed airstrip. But when the job was finished it'd been flattened into the runway and was mixed in with over 100 000 tonnes of fill from the quarry.

All the community got involved: farmers, townspeople, storekeepers, even the surfers. We worked rosters and shifts. Those that had to stay in their shops or businesses donated food or helped with morning tea. Anyone who hadn't brought any lunch along could get a free one at the local cafe.

Luckily there was no need for the Flying Doctor during the four weeks that the bulk of the work was done. Still and all, babies were born during that time. I'm not sure now if it was one or two. But something's for certain — with everyone working flat out I don't reckon that many would've been conceived.

Then after the job was completed there were two openings. The first was a political affair after some money had miraculously appeared out of government coffers to pay for the lighting and sealing of the airstrip. Not that we didn't appreciate it, mind you, but that opening was a fizzer in comparison to the second one.

The second opening was the real one. It was the one for the people. There was a true carnival atmosphere. Aircraft came from all over. There were fly-bys, lolly drops, parachutists, games and free gifts. We were just so proud of what we'd done that we had a special car sticker made up which read: WE BUILT AN AIRPORT.

Welcome to Kiwirrkurra

We've got a lot of Aboriginal people up here. They're great, the kids especially. They're so friendly and inquisitive. You get a lot of pleasure out of working with them. I love it.

Why just the other day I went over the Western Australian border to a place called Kiwirrkurra. We were picking up a woman who'd actually had a baby that morning and the baby was a little bit small so we were going to transport them both back to Alice Springs where we could keep a closer eye on things.

Anyway, we arrived a bit early.

Now I don't know if you've ever been out that way but the airstrips are just red dirt with spinifex growing along the side and a few sandhills around the place. And usually they have a little lean-to which is the 'airport terminal', so to speak, and this one had a little corrugated-iron lean-to. A real classic it is, all done up in the Aboriginal colours, with a sign which read:

WELCOME TO KIWIRRKURRA AIRPORT
900 FEET ABOVE SEA LEVEL
360 NAUTICAL MILES TO ALICE SPRINGS

I'd always wanted to get a photograph of the Kiwirrkurra 'airport terminal', so on this occasion I'd brought my camera along. So I took the photo. The next thing, the four-wheel-drive police vehicle turns up and there's about twenty kids in the back, on the top, all over the place, and they jump off and run over with their huge welcoming smiles.

'Hullo, hullo, hullo,' they're all saying.

'Oh, I've got my camera here,' I said. 'Do you mind if I take some photos of you all?'

Then they all push in front of the camera, and there's these twenty kids calling out, 'Just one of me only. Just one of me only.'

I didn't have that much film but I took a few photos anyway. Then I saw that one of the kids has a tattoo on his arm, you know, one of those lick-on tattoos.

'What've you got there?' I asked.

So he shows me. Then all of the kids lift up their shirts and they've got these tattoos stuck all over their stomachs and up their arms. Everywhere they were.

'Oh,' I said, to one of the kids, 'can someone take a photo with just me and you mob in it?'

'I'll take the photo. I'll take the photo,' said the oldest one.

Then he grabs the camera and starts clicking away

taking lots of photos. And all the kids want to be in on it. One jumps on one of my hips, another jumps on the other hip, and another kid stands behind me with her hands on my head. And they pack in tight around me. So there I am posing with these kids who are laughing and carrying on and I can feel something moving through my hair.

'Oh yeah,' I'm thinking. 'No worries, it's just that the kid behind me's playing with my hair.'

So we finished the photograph and I looked around at this kid, the one who'd had her hands on my head, and I noticed that she's not only got the most beautiful smile that you're ever likely to see but she's also got a half-melted Mars Bar dangling from her fingers.

Where's Me Hat?

We were flying out to Tibooburra to do a clinic one day when we received an urgent request to divert to Noocundra, in south-western Queensland. Someone had been severely burnt. The odd thing was, though, the chap who put through the call couldn't stop laughing. Naturally, we thought that it mustn't have been too serious, and we said so. But the chap, the one who was laughing, was adamant that the victim was badly burnt and, yes, it was anything but a laughing matter, which he was, if that makes any sense.

As the story unfolded, it'd been a stifling hot day in Noocundra and a few of the locals were in the pub attempting to escape the heat. The problem was that a large tiger snake was thinking along similar lines. It appeared in the pub and had a look around. But when it saw the accumulated gathering, it decided that it didn't like the company and headed off to the next best place it could think of, that being the outside toilet, one of those long-drop types. So out of the pub the tiger snake slithered, down the track a bit, into the outside toilet, and disappeared down the long-drop where it was nice and cool.

Now this chap saw where the snake had gone and he came up with the bright idea of incinerating it. He downed his drink, put on his hat, went and got a gallon of petrol, wandered back through the pub, down the track a bit, into the outside toilet, and tossed the fuel down the long-drop where the snake was. The problem was, after he'd tossed the petrol down the long-drop, he searched through all his pockets and couldn't find his matches. So he wandered back inside the pub.

'Anyone seen me matches?' he asked.

As I said, it was a very hot, still day in Noocundra, stinking hot, in actual fact. So after he found his matches, he thought that he may as well have another drink before he went back outside and sorted out the snake. Meantime the petrol fumes were rising up from out of the long-drop and, with there not being a breath of a breeze to disperse them, the toilet soon became nothing short of a gigantic powder keg.

After the chap had downed his drink, he grabbed his matches and put his hat back on. 'I'll be back in a tick,' he said. Then he wandered outside, down the track a bit, in the direction of the toilet. Without having a clue as to what he was in for, he walked into the toilet and took out a match.

'Goodbye, snake,' he said, and struck the match over the long-drop.

There are those from the outlying districts who go so far as to say that they felt the reverberations of the ensuing explosion. I don't know about that but, one thing's for sure, it certainly put the wind up the blokes who were hanging around the bar of the Noocundra pub. Such was the instantaneous impact of the blast that they didn't even have the time to down their drinks before they hit the floor. Mind you, that's only a rumour because, knowing some of the chaps out that way, no matter what the emergency they always finish their drinks before taking any action, even if it's a reflex action.

Still, you've got to feel sorry for the chap who went up in the sheet of flames. Critically burnt he was. Left standing over what had once been the pub's long-drop toilet with his clothes smouldering away. Stank to high heaven he did. It affected the chap's hearing too. Deaf as a post he was for a good while. And the shock, poor bloke. Even by the time we got there he was still as dazed as a stunned mullet.

As for his hat, it's never been found.

Whistle Up

A few years ago there were quite a lot of people moving into the pastoral country, out here near Meekatharra, in the central west of Western Australia. Anyway, being new to the area, they weren't familiar with the particular system we had if we wanted to activate an emergency call in at the Royal Flying Doctor base. Mind you, this is well before we had the modern transceivers. Back then, the emergency system was activated by a specially designed whistle. To give you some idea of this whistle, it was about three to four inches long and V-shaped, as in a Winston Churchill victory sign, so that you could blow down each side in turns, one long side, the other shorter.

So say, for example, there was an emergency. What you did was to press the button on the microphone which was attached to the radio then blow one side of the whistle for about ten seconds, then the other side for about six seconds, and that would activate the Flying Doctor emergency call in at Meekatharra.

Of course, it wasn't the perfect system. It definitely had its problems — it was rather difficult to activate the call signal in summer when you were competing against thunderstorms, or if you were one of the older folk or maybe a heavy smoker where you easily ran out of puff. And also, believe it or not, you had to develop a certain technique because when you changed from blowing down the long side to blowing down the short side you only had about a one second gap between blows otherwise it wouldn't work.

Anyway, the bloke who was the Base Operator in Meekatharra around this time decided that we should set a Sunday morning aside so that everyone could have a practice at blowing their whistles over the radio. Now this was a great idea because it not only gave a chance for the newcomers to get familiar with the system but it also provided the opportunity for those of us who'd lived in the area for a long time to brush up on our whistle-blowing skills.

So on this particular Sunday morning the Base Operator had us all raring to go. He got us on line then went through the rollcall to make sure that everyone was okay and that they had their special whistles nice and handy, which they did. After that was settled he began to go through the people one by one and listen to them blow their whistles, one long, one short. Quite a few people were successful, others had trouble. That was because they hadn't used the whistles before, or they ran out of wind or, in some cases, the whistles hadn't been used for so long that wasps or whatever had built little mud nests inside which prevented the whistles from working properly.

Anyway, the Base Operator got to this old fellow called Harry. Now Harry had been in the bush for quite a long time and the Base Operator said, 'Okay, Harry, now blow the long side of your whistle.' So Harry blew into his whistle and the sound it made came over our radios, nice and clear.

'Well done, Harry,' the Base Operator said, 'now blow the short side.'

Then Harry blew his whistle again and, oddly enough, it gave off the exact same sound. So the Base Operator asked Harry if he was sure that he'd blown down the other side of the whistle. Well, I can tell you that Harry sounded more than slightly put out by this remark. 'I most certainly did,' he snapped. 'I blew down one side of the whistle, then I blew down the other side of the whistle.'

That seemed clear enough, so the Base Operator then asked Harry just how long ago it'd been since he'd last used his whistle. Harry replied by saying that he couldn't really recall the exact date but it was definitely the year when a certain bush footy team took out the grand final.

'Well, okay then,' the Base Operator said, 'take your whistle and give it a good wash in some soapy water, then shake it dry, and I'll come back to you later and we'll give it another go.'

So off went Harry to wash his whistle and the Base Operator went on to listen to some other station owners blow their whistles, one long, one short. Then finally he returned to Harry. And when Harry blew his whistle, lo and behold, the shrill came across sounding exactly the same again, both the long side and the short side.

'Look, Harry, there's only the one tone coming through,' the Base Operator said. 'There must be something stuck down your whistle, maybe some mud, or wasps, or something like that. So how's about you go and get a little bit of wire and have a poke around inside.'

'Okay,' said Harry.

So away went Harry and when he got back on the air about five minutes later he tried his whistle again. There was no change. The result was the same. Still only one tone came through on both the long side and the short side.

The Base Operator by this stage was getting quite perplexed over the matter so he said to Harry, 'I can't understand what's going on here, Harry. There's definitely only one tone coming through. Are you dead sure that you're using the right whistle?'

'Of course I am,' replied Harry, 'it's the very same whistle I used when I was umpiring that grand final I told you about.'

Willing Hands

It was a Sunday. I was working an afternoon shift when we were called to a car accident at De Rose Hill, which is a cattle station just over the border into South Australia. Normally, Port Augusta would have taken it but for some reason they didn't have an aircraft available. That's why we went. We always help each other out. It's good like that.

From the information we received, a young tourist couple had rolled their car a few times and ended up crashing into a fence. The girl wasn't too bad, she only had a broken ankle, so after the accident she'd dragged the male occupant out of the passenger's seat and had laid him on the side of the road. Then while she was waiting for someone to come along she shielded the guy from the heat by holding a tarp over him.

But the guy was the big worry. We were told that he didn't have any body movement from his shoulders down.

Now De Rose Hill is a difficult place to land the twin engine aircraft because the airstrip's very short and it almost banks out onto the highway. So to gain every metre we could, we had to hit the airstrip as near to the road as possible. That meant while Pete, the pilot, kept his eyes glued on the strip ahead, I had my eyes peeled on the highway.

'Pete,' I'm saying, 'watch out for the road train on the left there.'

Anyway, we missed the road train, landed safely and checked the couple out. There hadn't been anyone medical there until the ambulance arrived, that's apart from some volunteers, of course, and they'd done a really good job. They'd put the guy on spinal boards and all.

Other than having broken her ankle, the girl was extremely distressed, so we gave her some sedatives then attended to the guy. The fifth vertebra in his neck, the C5, had actually gone over and severed his spinal cord. The C5 is above the C4. Christopher Reeves damaged a C4; you know him, don't you, the bloke who acted as Superman? That's why he lost his breathing capability and was placed on a life support machine. Luckily, this guy wasn't quite that bad. At least he could talk.

So we put drips and different things into the guy to get him as comfortable as possible. Now, he was a very tall man, extremely tall in fact, which made me even more thankful that there were so many willing hands there when it came to getting him onto a spinal mattress and into the aircraft. One old station chap even shaded the injured guy's face with his big bush hat. It was amazing just how helpful everyone was.

Now the way that the aircraft's set up is that there's a seat on the right-hand side, then room enough for two stretchers to go down the other side. But with the guy being so tall, we had to drag the spinal mattress up to the end of the aircraft and put his head on the seat so that we could fit the stretcher in with the girl on it. Then when she was settled we dragged the guy back down and put pillows and other bedding under his feet.

So finally we got the couple settled on board. 'Thanks,' we said to all the helpers. As I said before, they were fantastic. If it wasn't for them, we'd have been in big trouble. Anyway, we said cheerio to everyone, got into the aircraft and Pete started making his take-off preparations. Then just as we were about to taxi up the runway, a mob of cows came out of nowhere and wandered onto the airstrip.

By this time the ambulance people and our willing helpers had jumped into their vehicles and were on their way back to Marla or wherever, leaving no one behind to disperse the cows. So we taxied up and down a couple of times in an attempt to scare the cattle away. The only trouble was that by the time we reached one end of the runway, the cows had already wandered back onto the strip, down the other end.

We did have a telephone in the plane but that only worked within a certain radius of a few places and De Rose Hill wasn't within the radius of anywhere. So we had to go about it the long way.

What we did was we got in touch with the tower in Adelaide, who got in touch with the Adelaide Ambulance Service, who got in touch with the Ambulance Service in Marla, who got in touch with the ambulance that was returning from the accident scene, via a satellite phone, and they turned around and came back to shoo the cows off the airstrip, so that we could take off.

You Wouldn't Read About It

A good while ago they were filming that television show called 'Coopers Crossing' up here in Broken Hill. I mean, it's all over now but at the time they were aiming to shoot twenty episodes. The problem — or so I found out — was that they only had thirteen or so stories written. Now I reckoned that I had a great one to tell so I tried to get in contact with the girl who was involved in this particular incident, in the hopes that we could get together and collaborate on a script. The long and short of it was that I couldn't find her. Still can't. So perhaps if she ever gets to read this story she might like to get in touch. You never know.

Anyway, to go back a step or two, or three, before this particular incident occurred I used to work up at the mines in Broken Hill. That was until the day I received the old DCM. You know what that is, don't you? It's short for 'Don't Come Monday'. So, with a fair amount of time on my hands and nothing better to do, I hooked up with an operation driving a small tourist bus around the area.

Then one time we'd just made it into the tiny opal-mining town of White Cliffs before it bucketed down. I'd never seen anything like it. What's more, it left me with a big problem. See, I had some tourists on board who had to get back to Broken Hill by a certain day and there was no way that the type of bus I was driving could make it through in those sorts of wet and muddy conditions. Anyhow, as luck had it, I managed to organise their return with another carrier and I stayed behind with the bus.

So there I was the next day, stuck in the White Cliffs pub, waiting for the road to dry out. And with nothing much else to do, I filled in my day sipping on a beer, playing some darts, then having a game of pool, then some more darts, some more beer, a bit more pool, darts, pool, beer, and so on and so forth, until I wandered off to bed with the old wobbly boot.

It must have been about one in the morning when I was woken by the sounds of people running all around the place. Well, that certainly shook off the wobbly boot, I can tell you. Lights going on and off, cars taking off outside, shouting, the works. 'Christ,' I thought, 'the pub's on fire.' So I threw on some clothes and decided to get out of there quick smart.

The funny thing was though, as I was making my way outside it suddenly struck me that amid this confusion there wasn't even a whiff of smoke. So I pulled one chap over and asked him what all the kerfuffle was about. 'What the hell's going on?' I said. And this bloke told me there was a young girl who lived up the track at a station property, well, she'd been on a dialysis machine for a good while and the Flinders Hospital in Adelaide had just rung through to say that they'd found her a donor.

'But,' this chap added with a grim face, 'we've got to get her to Adelaide by 7 am, or else.'

Mind you, by this time it was just after 1 am in the White Cliffs pub which is way up in the north-west of New South Wales. What's more, the roads were almost impassable and they had less than six hours to transport the girl from the station property into White Cliffs and then fly her down to Adelaide, a distance of about 700 kilometres.

But none of that seemed to deter these people, the publican in particular. He was the nerve centre of the whole evacuation. He had all the radios and stuff and he was frantically organising things. The Flying Doctor at Broken Hill had been notified and was on the way up. One group of locals had gone to meet the father as he brought the girl into town through the floods. Another group had gone out to clean up the airstrip after the downpour and to set up the flares and get rid of the kangaroos.

To my eye they seemed to have a good enough handle on things so I wandered back to bed. Then in the morning I asked how the evacuation had turned out and I was told that they'd met the father out on the track, the plane had landed okay, they'd gotten the girl to Adelaide in time, and it looked like the operation in at Flinders Hospital was a success.

So that was that.

Then some time later, down the track a bit, I was taking a group of tourists around the Royal Flying Doctor Service base at Broken Hill. I was telling these people this story, about how they got the girl out of White Cliffs and into Flinders Hospital under some very extreme conditions and time constraints. There I was telling this story and one of the staff from the base pulled me aside.

'Guess what,' he said.

'What?' I replied.

'I was the pilot who flew that young girl down to Adelaide,' he said.

Well, that was one piece of coincidence.

Strangely enough, another happened about three years after that particular event. I'd left the small tourist operation by that stage and was working in the Adult Literacy Program in Broken Hill. Anyway, I got a call from a woman who said her grand-daughter was staying with her and she was having a bit of trouble with her writing. So I got together with this girl, a nice kid she was, and as always with these cases I made the comment, 'So, you've missed a little bit of school along the way, have you?'

'Yes,' she replied. 'I was on a dialysis machine for a while when I was living out on a sheep station.'

Well, that girl turned out to be the exact same girl who was picked up when I was stuck in White Cliffs all those years ago. You wouldn't read about it, would you?